MW00565890

THE LIFE POWER

AND

HOW TO USE IT

(1906)

Contents: Methuselah and the Sun; Three-Fold Being; Soul, Mind, and Body; How to Aim; The Substance of Things; The Spirit and the Individual; Crooked Paths; the Breath of Life; Affirmations and Wheels; Your Forces and How to Manage Them; Duty and Love; Will and Wills; Vibrations; Immortal Thought; God in Person; The Nobility; and more!

Elizabeth Towne

ISBN 1-56459-958-2

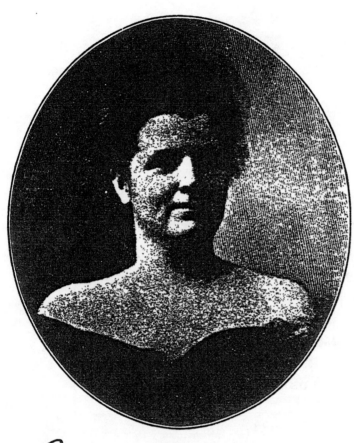

Cordially yours,
Elizabeth Towne.

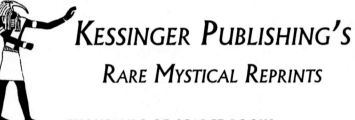

KESSINGER PUBLISHING'S
RARE MYSTICAL REPRINTS

THOUSANDS OF SCARCE BOOKS
ON THESE AND OTHER SUBJECTS:

Freemasonry * Akashic * Alchemy * Alternative Health * Ancient
Civilizations * Anthroposophy * Astrology * Astronomy * Aura *
Bible Study * Cabalah * Cartomancy * Chakras * Clairvoyance *
Comparative Religions * Divination * Druids * Eastern Thought *
Egyptology * Esoterism * Essenes * Etheric * ESP * Gnosticism *
Great White Brotherhood * Hermetics * Kabalah * Karma * Knights
Templar * Kundalini * Magic * Meditation * Mediumship * Mesmerism
* Metaphysics * Mithraism * Mystery Schools * Mysticism * Mythology
* Numerology * Occultism * Palmistry * Pantheism * Parapsychology
* Philosophy * Prosperity * Psychokinesis * Psychology * Pyramids *
Qabalah * Reincarnation * Rosicrucian * Sacred Geometry * Secret
Rituals * Secret Societies * Spiritism * Symbolism * Tarot * Telepathy
* Theosophy * Transcendentalism * Upanishads * Vedanta * Wisdom
* Yoga * *Plus Much More!*

DOWNLOAD A FREE CATALOG AT:
www.kessinger.net

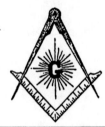

OR EMAIL US AT:
books@kessinger.net

TO WILLIAM E. TOWNE,

WHO HAS HELPED ME
			TO KNOW THE TRUTH,

I DEDICATE THESE PAGES.

The truth is large; no man hath seen the whole:
Larger than words; it brooks not the control
Of argument and of distinctions nice;
No age or creed can hold it, no device
Of speech or language; ay, no syllogism:
Truth is the sun, and reason is the prism
You lift before it; whence the light is thrown
In various colors; each man takes his own.
If this man takes the red as you the blue,
Is yours the whole? and is his truth not true?
Spirit is truth, howe'er the colors fall;
The fact comes back to spirit, after all.
                                    —Samuel Valentine Cole.

4

CONTENTS.

5

To see the beauty of the world, and hear
The rising harmony of growth, whose shade
Of undertone is harmonized decay;
To know that love is life—that blood is one
And rushes to the union—that the heart
Is like a cup athirst for wine of love;
Who sees and feels this meaning utterly,
The wrong of law, the right of man, the natural truth,
Partaking not of selfish aims, withholding not
The word that strengthens and the hand that helps!
Who wants and sympathizes with the pettiest life,
       And loves all things,
       And reaches up to God
       With thanks and blessing—
       He alone is living.
              —John Boyle O'Reilly.

I.

Methuselah and The Sun.

The sun gives forth to us heat and light rays, without which this old world could never be. Glory to warmth and light, which are power and wisdom shed upon us.

But there is likewise a third kind of ray shed by old Sol, whose mission we may not so readily bless. The sun's actinic rays are death-dealing. They cause disintegration, decomposition.

There are people who declare that time was when a great canopy of vapor hung over the earth and revolved with it, as Jupiter's vapory canopies now do; and that this vapory canopy kept off almost completely the actinic rays, while it admitted light and heat rays. Thus they account for Adam's and Methuselah's great ages. And they say that, unless this vapory canopy is again formed around our earth, to ward off these death-dealing rays, we shall never attain immortality in the flesh. They claim that as heat and light rays are power and wisdom, so the actinic rays are the Devil of the Bible, the Destroyer. And they believe that be-

7

fore man can be saved the Destroyer must be cast into outer darkness—shut out by that sheltering canopy of vapor.

An interesting and apparently plausible theory, is it not? But there are facts yet to be reckoned with. It is true that if a great watery veil spread itself over the earth to-day there might be no more death.

But neither could there be growth. Every form of life would continue as it is, wrinkles, gray hair and all. Why? Because there must be dissolution of old forms before there can be new ones made with that material. Take a photo plate as an instance: Here is a glass surface covered with a delicate gelatine; expose it in a dark-room under a red light and you can see just what it looks like; hold it there as long as you please and it still looks the same.

Now shut it into the black camera and sally forth on pleasure bent. The delicate film is undisturbed. But you come to a beautiful bit of woodland you want to "snap." You turn your focus upon it, and one little snap of a second's duration transforms that gelatine surface. Just for one instant of time you let in those actinic rays, and then all was darkness again inside the camera.

Now back you go into the dark-room and turn up the red light, by which you see again your beautiful bit of

8

woodland, reproduced on that delicate gelatine surface. If you let in a bit of daylight your picture would be gone in a wink—the delicate gelatine would be "pied" in an attempt to reproduce whatever it faced. But you don't let in the light of day; you "fix" your bit of beautiful woodland by dipping the plate in a solution which hardens the particles of gelatine to the glass.

Henceforth the light cannot affect that gelatine; the picture you have, but life, progress, change, possibilities, are gone from the delicate gelatine forever.

But if you could live forever under a red light you would not need to "fix" your negative; it would forever retain that picture. And if you continued to live under the red light you might as well throw away your camera and plates—you could never take another picture. And you wouldn't need such amusement either—not for long. A few days in the red light and you would be sick, and a few more days and you would go mad. Finally nature would "fix" you, and there would be no more change. (I wonder if scientists have ever tried keeping a dead form hermetically sealed under red glass. The cutting off of the actinic rays ought to arrest decay and facial change.)

You see, the actinic rays, the devil or destroying rays of the sun, are absolutely essential to all change in the photo plate. Probably the actinic rays soften and sepa-

9

rate the atoms of the gelatine, which are immediately polarized into the form of the scene it faces in the light and heat rays. Without the softening action of the actinic rays the gelatine could not take the form of the scene it faces; and without the light and heat rays it could not "see" and "feel" the scene, even if the actinic rays were present. It takes the trinity of rays, light, heat and actinic, to produce a photograph negative.

It is said that all inventions are but clumsy copies of mechanisms found in the human body and brain; that man contains on a microscopic scale all the inventions ever thought of, or that ever will be thought of. This is another way of saying that man is the microcosm, the universe the macrocosm. Victor Hugo expresses the same truth when he says "man is an infinite little copy of God."

The entire photographing process goes on in body and brain. Not a thought or sight but is photographed upon some tiny cell. Not a cell but may be cleaned of that impression, resensitized and given another impression.

Perhaps cells are immortal, as science claims. If so every cell must have undergone this cleaning, resensitizing and re-photographing process countless billions of times—with countless possibilities ahead.

And in every one of these picturings and repicturings

10

the actinic rays are utterly indispensable. So, I cannot believe that the immortality of anything but a marble statue is dependent upon the cutting off of the sun's actinic rays. To be sure the actinic rays cause dissolution; but dissolution merely precedes resolution; dissolution gives light and heat (wisdom and love-power) a chance to produce yet higher forms. Blessed be the destroying rays—blessed be nature's Devil; for he but clears the way for God himself, and cleans up and rearranges the rubbish after God has passed.

But when the race was in its childhood it looked upon the work done by these actinic rays, and fear was born. It saw things die; it saw destruction in the path of the wind; and like any child it imagined evil things. It personified the destroying power as Diablos, the Devil—which means destroyer.

It saw also the building, growing principle in nature and imagined a Builder.

But being a child it drew the childish conclusion that Destroyer and Builder worked eternally against each other, that they were enemies.

You see that was before the race had conceived the idea that two could work together; it was every man-savage for himself and the devil take the hindmost.

11

So the baby race began to love the Builder, God, and dislike and fear the Destroyer; and in its ignorance it personified both.

But here and there a clear-seer arose who glimpsed the truth. God spoke through Isaiah saying, "Behold, I make peace and I create evil; I, the Lord, do all these things." Solomon said the Lord "creates evil for the day of evil." And every seer of every Bible has tried to make clear the oneness, the all-wisdom all-power, all-presence of God.

All life is one. The sun is God manifest. The Destroyer belongs to the trinity and can no more be dispensed with than can the other two members, wisdom and love-power. And you may rest assured the Destroyer touches only that which needs dissolution that it may be transmuted.

Has anything gone out of your life? Have you lost that which you esteemed dear? Grieve not. It has been destroyed or taken away to make place for yet higher things.

God gives and God takes away in answer to your own highest desires. The Destroyer is but cleaning the plate for a more beautiful picture.

Be still and know that all things are working for the manifestation of your deepest desires. Work with things, not against them.

II.

Three-Fold Being.

Man is a three-strata being, instead of a two-strata one as Thomson J. Hudson theorizes. The obvious stratum is commonly called conscious or objective mind. This is the surface mind, the everyday mind, the mind we use in our waking hours.

Then there is the sub-conscious mind. The sub-conscious or subjective mind is the stratum of mind which receives the knowledge and wisdom which has passed through the conscious mind. The sub-conscious stratum of mind holds the habits and instincts formed at some time and place in and by the conscious mind. "Sub" means *under;* the sub-conscious mind lies *under* the conscious mind, as the depths of the lake lie under the surface.

But there is a third layer of mind which lies within and beyond both conscious and sub-conscious mind, and whose workings Hudson confounds with those of the sub-conscious mind. This may be called, for the lack of a better name, the super-conscious mind—the mind above conscious mind—the mind above consciousness.

13

This super-conscious mind is what we call God, out of which comes all wisdom.

Conscious mind is the point of contact between what we have already learned in this and previous states of existence, and the limitless reservoir of truth yet to be learned. Conscious mind is like unto the surface of a lake; sub-conscious mind is like the depths of the lake, every drop of which has at some time been on the surface, and is liable at any time to be recalled there; but super-conscious mind is like the rains of heaven and the streams from snow clad heights, whence the lake is perpetually replenished.

That which we already know, which we do by instinct, rests in the sub-conscious mind, ever ready to be recalled to the conscious mind. The conscious mind has to do with that which we are now learning. Super-conscious mind contains all wisdom, knowledge and power. In it we live and move and have our being and *from it we are able to call, by aspiration and inspiration, whatsoever we would know.*

The visible universe as it is, is the sub-conscious and conscious mind of God; it represents what has been thought out of the universal reservoir of truth. But it is only a taste of the wonderful supplies still awaiting our aspiration and inspiration.

Think of all the wonderful discoveries and inventions of the last sixty years—all *thought out* of that great universal reservoir; and eye hath not seen nor ear heard the glories that yet await us in the great super-conscious realm.

Mrs. Boehme illustrates individuality and solidarity by a star-shaped diagram. Each point of the star represents a person, a formed character; in other words, it represents the sub-conscious or habit self, the "nature" of the person. The center of the star represents God, the universal mind, with which every person is one on the unseen side. Looking at the points alone there is diversity, separateness; but looking from the center outward toward the points we see that points and center are all one, with no separating lines.

Now imagine a line cutting each point off from the center—an imaginary line, not a real one—and you will have a fair illustration of the conscious mind. The conscious mind lies between the personality and the universality of each of us; between the human and the divine of each; between what has been realized, and that limitless reservoir of beauties waiting to be realized.

Look at the star from the center and you will see that each point is simply a little bay projecting outward from the center; so each individuality is an inlet of God, each individual mind an inlet of divine mind.

And conscious mind is the imaginary line where personal mind and divine mind meet. You can readily see that one's conscious mind, then, would be filled with personality or divinity according as he looks down and is occupied with the "physical" being, or looks up and aspires toward the universal part of himself, the God part.

Now imagine the center of the star as being fluid, ever living and always free; and think of the points as being nearly solid, partially fixed. Imagine the points as containing water of life so muddy with false beliefs that it continually deposits along its edges layers of mud, ever hardening; with the water growing thicker and the beaches ever widening. Thus will you perceive the difference between personality and universality.

Now imagine the conscious mind endowed with will; note that when it turns toward the point of the star, toward the "material" part of itself, *it becomes tense with anxiety and thus shuts off the point from the center, preventing a free play of the currents of life through the star-point, the personality.* So the personality dries up, literally. This is the process by which we grow old.

Then imagine the conscious mind turned in faith and love toward the center of life—think, with this

16

broader vision and knowledge of life, how lightly it would hold the things of personality, of that little point of personality; knowing that the personality is only a little inlet of divinity, and that the broad opening between the two is always open, that personality exists as a result of ever-flowing currents of divinity, and that *only his own grasping and straining can hinder the currents;*—knowing all this, conscious mind turns away from the already realized personality and throws wide the opening into the great center of all life. Thus conscious mind looks up, not down; and comes into his kingdom of love, wisdom, power. This is inspiration and aspiration. Yes, you may receive what you will, provided you call upon the super-conscious mind, the One mind over all. Whatsoever you can ask this mind believing you receive, you shall have.

When you can't ask in faith it is usually because you have not dwelt enough with the thought of God, the divine self of all creation. When we dwell much in the thought of personality, things, "materiality," then God seems faint and far away and impotent, and we can't believe we shall receive what we ask.

We need daily periods for withdrawing from the physical life and dwelling upon the thought of our oneness with omniscience, omnipotence, omnipresence, and our oneness with each other. Thus does faith grow, aspiration and inspiration become our mental habit, and the waters of life flow freely through us.

The One Spirit will guide you in all the affairs of life, and you are "safe" only when following its promptings.

If you would know the spirit's leadings measure your impulses by the golden rule; for the spirit is Love to All.

III.

Soul, Mind, and Body.

If there is an individual soul that leaves the body at death, as most of us suppose, then this individual soul must be an organization of cell souls, just as the body is an organization of cells.

The body is referred to as the "shell," the "husk," the "house we live in," the "temple." In leaving the body, then, only the coarser elements are sloughed off and left as "dead," while the soul of every cell ascends, still organized in the individual soul; and the body cells disintegrate because the soul no longer holds them together.

This agrees with the statement of Theosophy that there is an "astral body" within the material body, which is like the material body but more beautiful. Many persons claim to have seen this astral body leave its "temple." Perhaps Paul meant this when he spoke of two bodies.

It seems reasonable to suppose that this spiritual body carries within it all knowledge gained in this state of being, and that in a new incarnation the older expe-

19

riences are "forgotten," just as a thousand things are forgotten every day of our lives—things which at some future time we may recall. The thing was there, in our sub-consciousness, all the time; it simply did not affect us strongly enough to make us think about it. A child's interest in this incarnation keeps in the background of sub-consciousness its memories of past lives. If it wanted to hard enough, and thought about it enough, it could recall incidents in previous states of existence just as it can recall an incident of yesterday or last year which it has temporarily forgotten.

Many people claim to have recalled past states of existence by desire and concentration, and many claim to have flashes of remembrance without any special desire or intention. And the Society for Psychical Research has on record many strange cases of dual or many-sided personality, etc., which seem to confirm this conception of soul and body.

It seems to me that the soul is the naked·life force which is one with spirit; that material experiences are the matrices by which the life force, or soul force, is formed and organized into individuality; and that we shed the "material" parts of the body as fast as we can—just as in the lower forms of life shells are discarded when backbones appear; the shell protecting and

moulding the life-form until it is sufficiently formed
and organized to do without the shell.

When the physical body becomes too stiff and un-
yielding a form for the growing mind or soul, then it
is discarded. And it looks as if the soul, through growth
and attraction, steps into a new incarnation where the
material at hand will afford it a better matrix.

As long as the body is alive and yielding, responding
readily to the developing organization of the individual,
the soul keeps changing in its matrix, its body, day by
day as needed; but a stiff, too-rigid and old-style matrix
or body has to be discarded in whole, for a new one.
"From the soul the bodye forme doth take," and when
the body becomes inadequate to express the soul growth
it is sloughed off altogether.

The body, astral and material, is the storage of the
past experiences and the wisdom organized through
those experiences.

The "objective mind," in the brain, is the surface of
this storage, the doorway by which all this wisdom and
knowledge entered into individual organization. The
brain is the switchboard by which we are able to use
this store of wisdom and knowledge at will.

The "objective mind" governs and directs not only
the switchboard, but all the sub-stores with which it
connects.

21

The "objective mind" also connects with the universal storehouse of wisdom, upon which it draws by what we call "intuition." It is through this connection with the universal that we are enabled to "rise higher than our source" of sub-conscious wisdom and knowledge gained in previous incarnations. In order to grow we need the super-conscious wisdom which is All.

Just as by desire and concentration we can recall the knowledge and wisdom gained in previous incarnations, so by desire and concentration directed toward the Universal, the Infinite, we call to us yet greater wisdom and knowledge than any yet realized.

The body which disintegrates after death is a mere collection of cell-cocoons from which the organized cell-souls have flown to new states of being. With its soul the body loses its feeling, the atoms disintegrating, each becoming what it was before, simply a bit of "dead matter" which is not dead at all.

The atoms of matter are just the same after death as before; but the organizing and informing spirit and soul, spirit or soul (for there is no dividing line between them), has departed, leaving each atom to live its little life again without relation to other atoms. Without this organizing spirit to draw and hold the atoms together they fall apart—"ashes to ashes."

The cell is the unit organization of the body, each cell

22

clothed with many atoms. The soul of the cell leaves it, just as the soul leaves the body as a whole.

That the astral body is an organization of cell souls, just as the physical body is an organization of cells, I have no present doubt.

And it looks reasonable to me to suppose that the soul, or astral body, carries within it all the records of all the individual's experiences since the beginning of time. That with every incarnation and experience this astral grows in wisdom and knowledge and beauty of character, I see no reason to doubt.

And by the power of universal attraction it is drawn in each reincarnation, to the exact parentage and condition it needs to help its growth in grace.

23

To Life, the force behind the Man, intellect is a necessity, because without it he blunders into death. Just as Life, after ages of struggle, evolved that wonderful bodily organ, the eye, so that the living organism could see where it was going and what was coming to help or threaten it, and thus avoid a thousand dangers that formerly slew it, so it is evolving to-day a mind's eye that shall see, not the · physical world, but the purpose of Life, and thereby enable the individual to work for that purpose instead of thwarting and baffling it by setting up shortsighted personal aims as at present. Even as it is, only one sort of man has ever been happy, has ever been universally respected among all the conflicts of interests and illusions. * * * I sing, not arms and the hero, but the philosophic man; he who seeks in contemplation to discover the inner will of the world, in invention to discover the means of fulfilling that will, and in action to do that will by the so-discovered means.

—Bernard Shaw:

IV.

How To Aim.

Without definiteness of aim nothing can be accomplished.

With too definite an aim very little can be accomplished.

This is the paradox of all accomplishment. It looks hard, but is in reality very easy—so easy that a child lives it.

The key to the problem is this: No man liveth unto himself and none dieth unto himself; we are all members one of another; all creation moves to "one far-off divine event," the definite details of which no human being has yet grasped. Perhaps none ever will grasp it. For how can the hand or the foot conceive the structure and purposes of the whole body?

There is a Universal Aim which includes and impels all individual aims. There is one great intelligence, one spirit, one purpose actuating every human being. The "Plan of Salvation" is not a mere superstitious myth. There certainly is a "plan," a "divine event," which we are all working at, whether we know it or not.

There is a Divine Ideal beckoning us every one. Glimpses of it are caught even by the fool who hath said in his heart there is no God, no oneness of life and purpose.

As our bodies are all members of God's body, so our ideals are members of the Universal Ideal; our aims are members of the Universal Aim.

Your hand may understand and define its impulse to grasp or release; but can it understand and define your aim and purpose, which gave it the impulse? We can imagine the hand understanding its own movements; but can it understand your movements and purposes? The hand says, "I want to grasp this"; but can it in any sense understand your purpose, which made it .want to grasp?

So you say, "I want to paint pictures." or "I want to make money,' or "I want to teach school," or "I want to be a home-keeper and mother," or "I want to build bridges." But can you tell why you want to do these things or others? Can you define the Great I WANT of which your *I want* is but an outcropping? Can you see the Universal Ideal of which your ideal is a detail? No; you can see your individual *I want,* but the Universal I WANT is too large for you to take in from your point of view.

Did you ever say to yourself, "I want to be a bridge

26

builder"; then after you had become a successful bridge builder did you find yourself rather disgusted with the bridge business? Did you find yourself saying, "I want to be a painter instead of a bridge builder"? And you couldn't imagine why your wants wouldn't stay satisfied with bridge building.

Can you imagine the hand being disgusted because after it had grasped the book awhile it found itself wanting to let go? Of course. The hand would not understand why it could not remain "constant" to its first desire: it would not see the reason for letting go.

So with us members of the "Stupendous Whole." Universal purpose and desire play through us. We know we "want" this and we "don't want" that. When we are on the "animal" plane we simply gratify our wants when we can, and are satisfied until another want impels us. By and by we begin to reason about our wants. We call some of them "good," and gratify them if we can. We call some of them "bad" and fight them with all our puny might—and are correspondingly unhappy. In both cases we fail to see why we want what we want.

When after we have learned to build bridges we find ourselves wanting to paint pictures we resist the desire and keep on building bridges. Then, if the Universal

27

Purpose really wants us to stop building bridges and make pictures it keeps on impelling us in the new direction until we finally find a way to get at the painting. If we are too stubborn the Universal I WANT gets us out of the way and raises up our sons and daughters to paint the pictures.

It is like this: In response to the Universal I WANT you have taught your good right hand to thread needles and sew, until it can almost do it in the dark. All the nerves and brains and muscles in your finger tips have learned that little trick. Now, in response to a new Universal I WANT, you decide that that good right hand of yours is to learn to run scales on the piano. You sit down at the piano, place your hand in position and impel it to strike the notes. But this sort of thing is entirely new to your fingers! Every little muscle is stiff, every nerve and every tiny bit of finger-brain protests that it can't run scales!—it does n't know how!—its work is sewing—it *can't*, so there! You say to yourself, "How stiff my fingers are, and how rebellious—they won't mind me at all!" But you keep on *sending your want, your will* into them. You "practice" long hours every day. And by and by you find your fingers have learned the new trick and can do it *without special thought and will from you.* You kept pouring your want into that hand until it became the hand's

28

want and will. From working against your want the
hand has come to work with it and by it.

Why did you do it? Because the Universal I WANT
kept pouring itself into you until you took up the practice; just as you poured the I WANT on into your
hands until they, too, wanted to do it, and did it.

Were your fingers extra rebellious? Did they fight,
and get tangled up, and imitate each other's movements? Then what did you do with them? *You kept
them at it;* and you kept them at it a great deal
longer time than you would if they had been more obedient fingers; you kept them practicing until they
learned to do the work willingly, with interest, artis-
tically. *Then* you gave them beautiful things to *play*
with, instead of hard things to *work* at.

Of course the beautiful things to play with are all
made up of the *very same* sort of things your fingers
have been *working hard* at. But the monotony of repetition is all gone from the beautiful play. It is joy to
play. It is "hard work" to practice scales.

*But without all those scales there can never be a sat-
isfying play.* In practice we learn by repetition to do
well and gracefully *one* thing at a time. In play we
string all these movements together in a satisfying play
of joy and praise.

We hope for the perfection of action which alone

29

makes satisfying play possible; therefore we keep practicing. The harder our fingers rebel the longer and more persistently we keep them at it—that is all.

Now the Universal I WANT keeps us at things in precisely the same way. The Universal is working out a glorious Ideal of perfect play, wherein every member of itself shall be shining, obedient, supple enough to play with grace and full joy the "music of the spheres." You and I being more or less stiff and disobedient and dense have to be kept at our practices until we learn to do them right. We say, "Oh, if I could only get into my right niche; but I seem to be held here in spite of all I can do!" We say we "don't like" the sort of "drudgery" we are "condemned" to—there must be something "wrong" with the universe, or with economic or family conditions, or we would not have to drudge at one kind of thing when we are "fitted" for something else, or want to do something else.

Our fingers cry out in the same way when we keep them at the scales—"Oh," they cry, "why are we compelled to this dreary commonplace repetition when our souls long for beautiful harmonies?"

You see, it never occurs to them that they are "compelled" to this commonplace scale practice *because* they long for beautiful harmonies and happy play. And it does n't occur readily to you and to me that we are held to our dish washing, our business routine, our bridge building *because* our souls long for greater things.

But it is so. The perfection of large ideals can never be attained except through perfection of detail; and through the dish washing, business routine, bridge building, we are perfecting the details of self-command, of body and brain control which will enable us to play the great harmonies our souls already feel.

The great things we feel and desire without being able to express them, comprise the Universal Ideal at which every soul is aiming, whether or not he knows it. The perfection of this great Ideal we seé as through smoked glass, darkly. We get all sorts of half-views of it, and spend a lot of time squabbling about it. But not one of us really knows even a tiny part of the glory and beauty and joy of that Universal Ideal, which includes and actuates all our personal ideals. "It doth not yet appear what we shall be." But we know that when the Great Ideal does appear we shall all have our places in the joy of its beauty, for every one of us will have had his place and done his part in working out that ideal.

The Universal Ideal is gently urging us on to ineffable good. But none of us can conceive the details of the good which is yet to appear. We are all hoping

31

and working for this "Indeterminate Good," as Hanford Henderson calls it. It constitutes our large Ideal, *which includes all our lesser, fleeting ideals and even our passing wishes and longings.*

It is with our large ideals that definiteness of aim is a mistake. An "indeterminate good" necessitates a general aim. It will not do to say "I know exactly where the blossoms will appear when the earth blossoms as a rose, and I know exactly the day they will appear; therefore will I till only those exact spots and get my ascension robes ready for that exact hour." The man who is so dead sure of his great aim will sooner or later, like "Perkins" in "Quincy Adams Sawyer," find himself perched on the ridgepole with his white robes flapping in the cold night and his goods in somebody's else possession. When one is too sure of the "far-off divine event" he muddles the present opportunity for hastening that event.

"Wisdom is *before* him that hath understanding; but the eyes of a fool are in the ends of the earth." The man who is too sure of the "indeterminate good" misses the present good. The man who aims at the Great Good which he cannot hit, misses the little Goods, near at hand, which need to be hit.

What should we think of a hunter who aimed only at big game beyond his gun's reach, while small game

32

gamboled at his feet? We 'd think him a fool who deserved to starve to death. Of course.

We miss our chances by straining after the big game beyond our reach.

The great ideal should have our faith, rather than our aim.

Aim only at that which is within reach, and trust the big things to time and the spirit.

You stand in the Now. Keep your aim for the things of the Now. Thus· will your aim gain accuracy and you will be ready for the Great Things when they shall at last appear in the Now.

Where are you Now? Are you building bridges? Then aim to build this one better than any other was ever built. Aim to improve your work now.

Aim to enjoy it all; for *only as joy brightens you can you see how to better your work and methods.*

And proficiency at bridge building means freedom to follow your next ideal. The greater your proficiency the nearer the top you get, and the more money you get for your work; and the more money you have the more time you can take for working out your next ideal.

In proportion as you are progressively proficient at your work your money stream will increase. In proportion as you enjoy your work you will grow in efficiency and money. The drudge is held to his work because he

· 33

does not put into it the love and interest and joy necessary to make him progressively proficient.

He says "lack of money keeps him from getting into a new line of work." That is it exactly—the Universal Spirit which urges us on keeps the money away from us until we have gained in this thing the proficiency needed to fit us for other work.

Are you building bridges and at the same time aiming to paint pictures? And are you too poor to drop the bridge building and devote all your time to painting pictures? Then I say unto you have faith in your desire to paint pictures, for your desire is an outcropping of Universal Desire and is certain to find its satisfaction. Your desire is the desire of Omnipotence, Omniscience, which will in no wise disappoint itself. All desires shall be fulfilled in the fullness of time.

Would you hasten the time? Then have faith in your desire; but aim at the bridge building. Do better and better the work you find to do until the way opens to a new line of work.

And do every detail of your bridge building as if it were the painting of the greatest picture. Think you that accuracy of observation, delicacy of touch, harmony of thought and power of expression are gained only by dabbling paint on a canvas with a camel's-hair brush? No. Bridge building has its place in training

34

a great painter. Put your soul into it while you are held to it, and give it its full chance to do the work.

Have faith in your desire to paint pictures, but aim your energies at the bridge you are building now. Keep your faith high, your aim true, and verily in an hour when you least expect it the way will open from bridge building to picture painting.

Where are the cowards who bow down to environment—
Who think they are made of what they eat, and must
*   conform to the bed that they lie in?*
I am not wax,—I am energy!
Like the whirlwind and waterspout, I twist my envi-
*   ronment into my form, whether it will or not.*
What is it that transmutes electricity into auroras, and
*   sunlight into rainbows, and soft flakes of snow into*
*   stars, and adamant into crystals, and makes solar*
*   systems of nebulae?*
Whatever it is, I am its cousin-german.
I, too, have my ideas to work out, and the universe is
*   given me for raw material.*
I am a signet, and I will put my stamp upon the molten
*   stuff before it hardens.*
What allegiance do I owe to environment? I shed
*   environments for others as a snake sheds its skin.*
The world must come my way,—slowly, if it will,—but
*   still my way.*
I am a vortex launched in chaos to suck it into shape.
*   —Ernest Crosby.*

.V.

The Substance of Things.

"To a certain extent I have been benefited by these teachings. In some ways they do not appear to have a very practical
result. It is possible to concentrate and obtain small things, but
any real change of surroundings seems to be quite dependent
upon circumstances entirely outside my own will." H. B.

Thus writes a shortsighted and faithless one—faithless because of her shortsightedness. Another woman
who has observed the same things writes thus: "If I
see no great results now *I know it is because I am working for large things.*"

Life "concentrates" on a mushroom and grows it in
a night; but an oak requires twenty years of "concentration." A woman "concentrates" on a good dinner,
a bit of sewing, the control of her tongue for an hour,
$5.00 for a new hat, the cure of a headache, and suc-
cess crowns each effort. These are little things, the
mushrooms of an hour, used shortly and soon forgotten.

The same woman "concentrates" for a complete
change in disposition or environment, for anything in
fact which seems a long way off from present conditions.
Now, if she is a shortsighted woman she has little or

37

no faith in anything which she cannot see, hear, taste, smell or feel. She can see, taste and smell a mushroom, so she believes in it. She could see an oak and believe in that. But she cannot see the acorn growing underground, therefore she has no faith that there is an oak growing. And if there is already a little oak in sight she cannot see it grow, no matter how steadily she looks at it; therefore she "fears" the oak is not growing.

But the far-seeing woman is different. She sees *through* things. She feels the intangible. She hears, smells, and tastes that which moves upon the face of the deep and brings forth *things*. She touches the true substance (that which *stands under*) of things which are to be.

Her faith rests in invisible life; the other woman's faith rests only in the visible things which life has made.

To say that H. B. has no faith would be an untruth. Every living being is full of faith, or he could not live. Faith is in the atmosphere and we live by using it, just as a fish lives by using the water. Faith springs eternal in every human breast, fed from the universal source. To talk of one's little faith or one's much faith is like talking of the earth's squareness.

Every soul lives by faith and plenty of it. But he

38

lives by faith in what? There's the rub. Until we emerge from a sense of materiality—and no one has as yet got more than his nose above these muddy waters—we live by faith in things seen, smelt, tasted, heard and felt. These are the only things we are familiar with; to them we pin our faith, and pride ourselves upon our good sense, reason and lack of "superstition." "I can't believe in anything unless I can see it," is our self-satisfied cry; "you can't fool me with your religious hocus-pocus, nor with your rabbit's foot and horseshoe and four-leaved clover; I can see no connection between a rabbit's foot and your good luck, therefore I know no connection exists; I can see no big God on a great white throne, consequently I know none exists; show me your God; show me the string which connects the four-leaved clover to your good luck and I'll put my faith in it."

The material one reckons without his Unseen Host. By and by the Unseen begins to juggle with him. His beautiful plans, every step of which he could plainly see, are blown awry. He can't see why! The things in which he had such faith begin to totter and tumble about his ears. He can't see why! Reluctantly he begins to see that there are mighty forces he can't see. His whole beautiful material world begins to dance to strings he can't see!

Ah, so there are things he can't see, hear, smell, taste or feel! They may be a fearful and chaotic jumble; they seem to be; but they are there, after all his certainty that he could see, smell, hear, taste and feel The Whole Thing.

And he begins to reach out toward these unseen things. He peers and peers into the darkness and stillness. And as he peers his faiths gradually loosen their hold upon the old visible things and begin to reach out into the darkness and silence. He sends his faiths groping, groping, feeling their way through the Invisible, always seeking the strings to which visible things have been dancing and tumbling.

At first all is darkness; but by and by faith gets its tentacles around Something Unseen;—ah, there is Something which disposes what man proposes—an unseen, untasted, unheard, unsmelt, unfelt Something. A terrible Something it may be, but still a Something, all-powerful, all-present. He has sent his feelers into the Invisible and touched God, the soul, the life-principle, which makes and unmakes, gives and takes away all those little things to which he was wont to pin his faiths.

The next thing is to find out the nature of this mighty Something whose home is in the Invisible. But how find out the nature of the Unseen? Not by touch,

40

taste, smell, sight or hearing—not at first anyway. But by its fruits you may know a tree to be good or bad. By its fruits you may know the invisible powers to be beneficent or malefic. And the material one is familiar with fruits, with things. He built such beautiful things himself, so he ought to be a judge of the fruits of labor. The fruits of his labor were all good, he knows they were. If only the great Unseen had not spoiled them all! Oh, the labors of the Unseen brought his own good efforts to naught—the Unseen must be a terrible and evil power; its fruits are destruction of his own good buildings. He fears this Great Unseen Power to which his faiths are beginning to pin themselves.

But wait: Good is beginning to rise from the ashes of his ruins. This so terrible calamity is turning out a blessing! New and greater things are forming, to take the places of the lost fruits! And they are good. Oh, this Great Unseen works in terrifying mystery but its fruits are good.

Now he is ready to "come unto God." He begins to see the un-seeable things, and his faiths tendril them.

Those who would "come unto Him must believe that He is, and that He is a rewarder of them that diligently seek Him."

Those who would understand and feel and use the

41

invisible forces must believe that they are, and that they reward those who diligently seek to understand and use them.

The Unseen things move the visible world. The material one being pinned by his faiths to the things of the world is moved as the world is moved. He is a mere puppet in the hands of the Unseen powers.

As he looses the faiths which bound him to the world rack, and sends his faith tendrils into the Unseen, he becomes one with the powers which pull the world-strings.

"Faith is the sub-stance (the underlying and creating principle) of things hoped for, the evidence of things not seen."

The material one's faith is pinned to things already seen; therefore his creative principle is poured into the thing already created.

Then Life juggles and tumbles things until the material one's faiths are torn loose from their material moorings, and go feeling out into the Unseen for new things to cling to. When the whole bunch of visible things has failed us; when houses, lands, money, friends, and even fathers and mothers and brothers and sisters have gone back on us, what is there left to pin our faiths to? And without something to have faith in how could we live at all? We couldn't live without faiths to

42

steady us; witness the suicides and the deaths from broken hearts.

And if all visible things have failed us, if our faiths are broken loose from fathers, mothers, brothers, friends, houses and lands, where else can our faiths take hold again except in the region of the Unseen?—the region where "the wind bloweth whither it listeth and thou canst hear the sound thereof but canst not tell whence it cometh nor whither it goeth," the region of substance, of creative power.

It seems very terrible to have our faiths broken loose from fathers, mothers, brothers, friends, houses and lands; but it is good for us, as time always proves. Broken loose from the effects of creative energy our faiths reach out into the Unseen and tendril the very energy itself. From a state of oneness with things we evolve a new being at one with the creative power within things.

What are the unseen things to which our torn faiths begin to attach themselves? Our faith itself is unseen, the sub-stance of things hoped for, the substantial evidence of things not yet seen.

What do we hope for that we have not yet seen? First of all we hope for peace—another of the substantial unseen things. We hope for love, the most substantial of unseen things. Oh, if we had but peace

43

and love we could count all else well lost! And behold, by unseen faith tendrils our bruised faiths attach themselves to the unseen substance of peace and love. Wisdom is an unseen substance—our unseen faiths attach themselves to the unseen source of wisdom. Thought is unseen; our faiths, torn loose from things, begin to reach out into the unseen realm of thought. Ideals are unseen things. Our faiths, torn loose from the already-realized, begin to tendril the unseen ideals, the race's ideals, the family ideals, and lastly our individual ideals.

Our unseen faiths become one with these unseen ideals; and through these little faith tendrils we begin literally to draw the ideal down into our physical being and out into the visible world. Through our faith tendrils the ideal is literally ex-pressed, pressed out into visibility.

When our faiths were attached to material things, the material things being negative to us, sucked us dry. Now our faith tendrils reach upward to the unseen ideal realm of real substance, to which we are negative, and by the same law of dynamics it is we who draw the life; draw it from the unseen realm of real life substance.

Of ourselves we could do nothing—the things to which our faiths attached us sucked us dry of power, and the unseen powers finally tore us loose; but now

44

that we are tendriled by our faiths to the Unseen, "the Father" in us and through us doeth the works of rightness that bring peace.

And behold, we are filled with the unseen power, and through our faith in the Unseen we pass on the fruits of the spirit, which are "love, joy, peace, longsuffering, gentleness, meekness, faith, temperance."

And being filled with the power of the Unseen we pass on the fruits of the spirit to fathers, mothers, brothers, friends, houses, lands; pass it on in every act of life and in every breath we take. We *breathe out* that which, through our faith-tendrils, the Great Unseen *breathes into us.*

Then, behold, that which is written comes to pass: "*Ye shall have an hundredfold more houses and lands and fathers and mothers and brothers in this present time.*" You shall have them to use at will.

While you were *attached* by your faiths to things *they* used you; now you use them.

Pin your faiths to the Unseen things and let patience have her perfect work. So shall you realize your heart's full desire. Let things rock as they will; let facts be stubborn and conditions hard if need be. Never mind them. To mind them is to pin your faiths to them.

Mind the Unseen things. Pin your faiths to your ideals.

Flout facts and hard conditions!   Believe in the Unseen.

Train your faiths upward.

"Whatsoever ye desire *believe that ye receive*," and
you shall surely have it.   If it is a mushroom expect it
in a night.   If you desire a great oak give it time to
grow.   In due time, perhaps in an hour when you least
expect it, it will surely appear.

The one thing needful is to pin your little faiths to
the Unseen Source of all things.

Believe in the great unseen part of yourself and the
universal.

VI.

To Get at the Substance.

All desirable and as-yet-unexpressed things are in the silence waiting to be drawn into expression through aspiration and inspiration.

Of course one can aspire and inspire anywhere and under almost any conditions. I remember one great aspiration of mine which was satisfied whilst I was sitting in a crowded street car with folks standing in front of me and others clinging to the running board.

The Things of the Silence are everywhere present, permeating solid things as the X-rays do. All creation cannot hinder a man communing with the Unseen at any time and in any place—all creation cannot hinder him except as he lets it.

But that is the trouble—he lets it interfere unless he is in almost agonizing earnest about the unseen things. That momentous hour on the crowded street car came after weeks of most earnest "seeking," after weeks of almost constant "concentrating" on this one thing I wanted to receive from the Unseen. I was so absorbed

47

in that one subject that the crowds were as nothing to me.

In order to get anything—wisdom, power, love—from the silence one's whole interest must be absorbed in the matter.

Your interest is like the plate in a camera; it receives impressions only from that upon which it is turned. And the camera must be held steadily in one position until the impression is received.

The human camera receives impressions from the unseen in exactly the same way that it receives impressions from the seen world.

But it takes a longer time to receive a complete impression from the unseen, just as it takes a longer time to get a good negative in the dark.

The unseen is the dark to us; hence the long time it often takes to get a complete impression of anything we desire to receive in the silence. It takes a longer "exposure" to get the impression.

"Concentration" is merely the steady "exposure" of the attention, the interest, to the thing we desire to realize, to make tangible.

Now the busy person, the person who is interested in a thousand things, keeps his interest so busy taking instantaneous photographs that he has no time to get impressions from the unseen. His mind is constantly

48

flitting from one thing to another. When it happens
to turn toward the unseen it simply sweeps the dark
quickly and comes back to earth again without an impression.

Instead of a steady aspiration toward the ideal there
is a constant perspiration toward the real.

As there is nothing new under the sun the only progress made is around and around the same old things.

The only real relief from things as they are lies in
the unseen.

The only way to get at the relief is to "concentrate"
on the unseen things. In order to do this the attention
must be called away from seen things. The mind must
be "set on things above," and kept set until the "renewing" is complete.

People who are not yet satisfied that the visible world
does not and cannot satisfy, will see no need of going
into the silence on set occasions. And there is another
class who are apt to see no need of it—the class whose
"concentration" on the invisible is so constant that
material things assume the subordinate relation. These
are people who have "got the truth" by coming up
through great tribulation; who have run the gamut of
things and found the principle behind things.

And almost invariably, if not always (I have never

heard of an exception), these are people who have tried nearly every method of spiritual culture extant, have practiced fasting and prayer, breath exercises, denials and affirmations, and treatments and concentrations of every conceivable kind.

Martin Luther was one of these; and at last, when he had tried everything else and was crawling up the church steps on all fours, he "found the truth." Immediately he arose, repudiated all his good works as unavailing, and went about praising and preaching that not by works but by faith we are healed.

Eight or ten years ago I heard Paul Militz, who had worked for years at all manner of spiritual, mental and breath exercising, repudiate it all as "unnecessary." "Not any of these things avails you," he said. And others who have "found the truth" reiterate the same statement.

And yet every one of them has "found the truth" through those very practices.

If Martin Luther had stopped short of crawling up those church steps as his own seeking spirit bade him, he would never have "found the truth." If Militz, Shelton, Burnell, *et al.*, had left out one of their practices they would still be "seeking."

The spirit in every man bids him do things and refrain from doing other things, in order to "save" himself from something or other. Is this universal urge only a lie? No.

These concentration exercises are kindergarten methods by which we learn to use ourselves. When by practice we have learned how we discard the kindergarten methods. What was gained by self-conscious effort becomes habit. We turn intuitively to the unseen, whereas we used to turn to it only by conscious effort, by special practices.

But why repudiate the practices? Why tell others who are trying to learn how, that their efforts are all useless? By practices we found the way; why discourage practice?

There are people who as yet are wrapped up in the material. There are those who are wrapped up in the unseen. Neither of these are in present need of set times for "concentrating" upon the unseen, the ideal side of life.

But there is a third great "middle class" who are not absorbed in the already manifest world, and who want to be one with the unseen world of causation. To these I say, follow the example of all the "adepts" of all the ages; practice "concentration."

To all who want to accomplish something I say, Go into the silence regularly for power and wisdom to accomplish.

51

To those whose interests are mainly in the material world, but who want to understand and be deeply interested in the unseen world—from whence come all things,—to those I say, Go into the silence at regular periods every day.

To all humanity who are longing for Something, I say, All things are in the Silence; be still and know.

VII.

The Spirit and The Individual.

"I was washing my breakfast dishes one morning when it occurred to me to go to visit a friend who lived several miles away. I did my work and started to dress for my journey, when there came over me such a feeling of depression, or despondency, or gloom, that I could not understand. I kept on getting ready, all the time trying to reason away the feeling. But it would not go. Finally I got my hat on and one glove and started for the door, when such a heaviness came over me that I turned back into my room and sat down saying, 'God, I want to know what the meaning is of all this.' The answer came loud, strong and firm, 'Stay at home.' I stayed, and taking off my hat, gloves and cape I felt so light I seemed to walk on air. At the time I supposed the voice (I call it voice for want of a more definite term) had told me to stay at home because some one was coming to me for help. This was my first year as a teacher and healer. But not a soul came that day, nor that night, and the thought flitted through my mind that perhaps it was all nonsense after all and I might as well have gone. Well, the outcome was that the train I would have taken met with a fearful accident in which many were killed or badly injured. This is only one of many similar experiences I have had. I do not stop to reason out things. The world has tried for 1900 years to follow reason, and look at the outcome. I follow my intuition and it never fails me."—Flora P. Howard, *Los Angeles, Cal.*

One's reason is not a thing to be belittled and denied. It is his crowning glory, created for use.

But it is not all the wisdom a man has access to, nor is it the greatest. The man who exalts his understanding above the wisdom of the rest of creation, *and un-creation,* is a fool and sure to come to grief.

But he who rejoices in his personal understanding or reason as the means by which he taps the source of all wisdom, is in a fair way to profit by his own intelligence and the universal intelligence besides.

Everybody knows his foresight is not so good as his hindsight. He has demonstrated the fact many a time, by as many little tumbles off his high horse. Really, it seems as if he might have learned by this time not to be quite so sure about his reason.

After Mrs. Howard knew that the train she meant to go on had been wrecked she saw, plainly, why it was unwise for her to go on that particular train. Her reason had been enlightened, her hindsight perfected.

By what? By universal intelligence. Suppose New York city should set itself up as the center of all wisdom—suppose she were to say, "What I cannot reason out is not worth knowing." Suppose she continued to send out decrees into all the world, but turned up her nose at the messages sent in to her. What do you suppose would happen? She would go to smash in a week. It is by her reception of all those messages as to outside doings, that she is enabled to reason out her business problems and send out messages that move the

54

world. To exalt New York knowledge and reason, and despise outside knowledge and reason, would quickly ruin her.

Intuition is the wireless line by which we receive directions from every other station in the universe. After Mrs. Howard had received and obeyed her message from the universal—some days after—she knew why she had been so directed.

He who is puffed up in his own conceit is eternally despising his intuitions, following his back-number reasons, and getting into the "accidents." Then he wonders why he is so abused.

You see, we have none of us ever passed this way before. This day is a new day; this bit of road has never been traveled before. Nobody can know by reason what we shall run into just around the bend there. He may make a rough guess at it, but he cannot know.

But—there is Something which, whether it knows or does not know consciously, what is, or will be, around that corner there—there is Something which can and does send us by the wireless line a message to keep away, or to go to it, as the case may be.

Now Mrs. Howard was a woman with no desire to be in such a smash, and she believed her intuitions would keep her warned away from them.

Now next door to Mrs. Howard there may have lived

55

another woman, just as "good" as Mrs. Howard, just as devoted to her intuitions, who received a message to go on that train. At the same moment Mrs. Howard's heart grew heavy and she heard the message, "Stay at home," this other woman's heart grew light and she heard the message, "Go." So she went blithely forth to the train. She mounted the steps and walked into the car and along past several vacant seats before she felt the impression to sit down. She sat down and gazed happily out of the window.

By and by, as they were bowling swiftly along there came a sudden crash, and shrieks, and hiss of steam. Then there was work to do.

This woman neighbor of Mrs. Howard's, beyond a little shaking up from which she almost instantly recovered, was entirely uninjured. There were dead and dying in front and behind her, but she was safe. There was work to do and she was there to do it.

You see, this woman was a physician and surgeon, and the only one on the train. She had been years preparing for such work, and she believed her intuitions would lead her, strong and well herself, into just such opportunities as this. So the message which depressed Mrs. Howard brought light to the soul of this woman.

Each received and interpreted the message according to her own particular character.

And what about the injured and killed? They too were "led by the spirit." Each by his own self-built character related himself to his particular "fate." I wouldn't wonder if a good many of them did it by filling up on the accident and criminal columns of the daily papers. The man who thinks in terms of accident is pretty sure to meet them. But probably more of the "victims" were drawn through their false religion. The man who thinks himself (who really thinks it, "in his heart")—who thinks himself a "vile worm" and a great sinner deserving of a "bad end," and yet who has not "repented," is daily relating himself more closely to all sorts of violent and horrible things. And everywhere and at all times the violent man, the strenuous man, no matter how "good" he may be, is preparing himself to be led into whatever catastrophe fits him. There is no hit and miss about our "fates"—we get just what we are fitted for.

And through all ages we have been fitting ourselves; and we are still at it. He who is not busy fitting himself for the best is relating himself to the less good. He who fits himself to die with his boots on will die so. He who fits himself for "accidents" will die by an accident. He who fits himself for life may perchance never again see death.

When the bubonic plague is about to appear in a

57

place all the birds fly away. What warned them? Oh, that was only "instinct"—something common, that we wise beings never use.

Before Mt. Pelee spit destruction, all the wild animals (not one of which could have had any personal knowledge, or any record of volcano lore) fled from the vicinity. The tame animals whimpered and cowered and those which could ran away. Then the people's hearts began to sink and the most ignorant of them ran after the animals. As Mt. Pelee grew more emphatic in her prophecies all hearts grew heavier and heavier and all souls heard the message "Go." Then there was hurried preparation for a hasty exodus. But no; the wise, educated, sensible men put their heads together and decided that they would not and others should not be guided by any such common thing as "instinct," or by their own sinking hearts. No! Even though their hearts fell into their shoes and their knees knocked and their teeth chattered they would be sensible, they would; they'd use their divine reason, they would—Mt. Pelee had never destroyed them before and it would n't now.

So the wise reasoners corralled the poor fools. And they were well corralled. Only one ever got away.

Now just what this spirit is like that tries to lead us into all truth, is a thing I don't know. But that there is such a spirit that pervades and would save all creatures

58

from harm I do know, both by intuition (the spirit's witness with my spirit) and by actual and repeated experiences of both kinds. I have been led of the spirit into ways of pleasantness, peace and plenty; and before that I turned up my nose at the spirit and went my own way into all sorts of troubles.

And I have a theory, based on the spirit's witness with mine, as to what this spirit is and how it acts. The spirit is the universal intelligence which fills this universe so full there is not room for anything else. There are just little eddies and whirls and currents and cross-currents in this great ocean of intelligence. And you are one eddy in it, and I another; and each of us sets up little swirls and currents that move us about and move other things to us. And when a leaf floats by it is drawn into our eddy, but when we swirl by a rock, the rock is unmoved and so are we. We are not related to the rock.

When gold is placed beside a horseshoe magnet it stays put. The magnet and gold are not interested in each other. But that does not prove that the magnet is stupid and dead. No, there is a great current of longing in that magnet. If it had means of locomotion it would go about the world seeking, seeking—perhaps never knowing just what it was seeking, but still seeking. And by and by it would begin to feel a definite

59

inclination to go in a certain direction. Now if it is just a fool magnet without great pride in its brains it will follow that definite inclination. And as it journeys the drawing power will grow, and it will journey faster, and behold, it will fly into the arms of its affinity, a steel bar. And it will cling and cling, and the bar will cling, and joy will be born.

It takes two, and an exchange of intelligence, to bring joy into being.

Or perhaps our magnet will stay at home and long, long, until it draws to it steel filings.

This is not so fanciful as you may suppose. All things are intelligent. All things are putting their little compulsions on all creation for satisfaction. And in due time all compulsions will be met. The great sea is seething with intelligence, and affinities are coming together.

It is the attraction of the magnet for the steel that constitutes what I call the spirit. That attraction is intelligence.

When in doubt as to the meaning of your solar center feelings, do nothing. Come back as Mrs. Howard did, sit down; be still; ask for the meaning; and obey.

VIII.

By Crooked Paths.

The Rev. R. F. Horton tells a little story of a remarkable answer to prayer. He was with a party of tourists in Norway. In exploring some wild and marshy country one of the ladies lost one of her "goloshes." The overshoe could not be replaced short of Bergen, at the end of their tour, and it was out of the question to attempt to explore that wild country without rubbers. The golosh must be found, or the tour curtailed.

As you may imagine, every member of the party set diligently to work to find the missing rubber. Over and over they hunted the miles of glades and mountain sides they had traversed. At last they gave it up and returned to the hotel.

But in the afternoon a thought came to Dr. Horton —why not pray that they find the shoe? So he prayed. And they rowed back up the fjord to the landing of the morning, and he got out and walked directly to the overshoe, in a spot he would have sworn he had before searched repeatedly.

I remember a similar experience of my own. There

61

were four of us riding bicycles along a rather sandy road some distance from town. Two were spinning along on a tandem some distance ahead of us, on a down grade, when a rivet flew out and the chain dropped. The tandem ran for a quarter of a mile on down the hill and slowed up on the rise beyond, so that our friends were able to dismount without injury.

By this time we had overtaken them, having ridden in their track, and learned for the first time the cause of their halt. Of course everybody's immediate thought was, "Oh, we can never find that tiny gray rivet in this gray dust—probably the other bicycles ran over it—and home is three miles off!" But we all retraced our steps, diligently searching. Two of the party are crack shots with the rifle, with very quick eyesight. I thought one of these two might find the rivet. But we all walked slowly back, far beyond the point where they became conscious of their loss, and no one spied the rivet.

Then it occurred to me that the high spirit within had not been called to our assistance. Immediately I said to myself, "Spirit, you know where the rivet is!— please show it to me!"

I thought of the spirit as the Law of Love or Attraction, which is the principle of all creation, and instantly the idea came that the little rivet could attract the eye's

62

attention if the eye were willing to be attracted. These words floated into my mind, "Rivet, rivet, rivet my eye!"

By this time I had fallen behind the others. So I walked leisurely, calmly along, eyes willing, and those words saying themselves over and over in my mind.

And the rivet riveted my eye! I, who considered myself very slow of sight, found the rivet. And I know it was because I turned to the universal self, to God, to the Law of Attraction for the help needed, for the knowledge which not one of us had in consciousness, but which was certainly present in the universal mind in which we live and move and have our being.

Just the other day I had a little experience which illustrates the "man's extremity is God's opportunity" idea. For years I have said I could never find ready made garments to fit me. Have tried many times; waists all too short and narrow in front, sleeves skimpy. But I keep trying, every year; for everything is evolving you know, even clothes and tailors.

I wanted a new white lawn shirt waist and wondered if I couldn't find one ready made. Tried in the biggest suit house in Springfield; no good. Then one day I had an impulse to try the best places in Holyoke. One or two almosts, but nothing that would quite do. Gave it up.

Then I had another impulse to try a store of which I have always said, "I never found there anything I wanted." I nearly passed the store, saying to myself, "No use to try there, and it is late anyway." But there came the thought, or rather impression, that the spirit impelled me and I would better go. "We'll see if it is the spirit," I said to myself—"I believe it is." It was. I found the waist I wanted, and I found a pretty white lawn suit besides! In the most unlikely corner in the vicinity, according to my judgment and experience.

There is a little law in here that I want you to notice. *The spirit leads us through impressions or attractions; and it is limited in its revelations by our mental make-up, which is the conscious and ruling part of us.*

Why did not the spirit impress me in the first place to go to that store, where that waist and dress had been waiting for me since spring? And I had wanted them since spring. The spirit did impress me about it, but when the spirit said *"shirt waist"* to me I said, *"Springfield*—if they have n't a fit there they won't have it anywhere; and anyway I *know* I'll never find it." But I tried—*without faith*. That shut the spirit up for the time.

But at the very first opportunity, on the first afternoon when I was n't too busy to even think about such things, the spirit whispered "shirt waist" to me again.

64

And I did n't let the spirit get any farther with its impressions; instead of asking the spirit where to go for a shirt waist I said, "Oh, yes, shirt waist—of course—I 'll go to A.'s and B.'s and C.'s, where I generally get other things that suit me."

You see, my habit mind, preconceived opinions, again settled the matter. It was not until I had given up finding anything at these places, and was going right by the door of the other store, that the spirit had a chance even to whisper its name to me. The spirit had to lead me around all my prejudices in the matter, before it could get me to think of that place. My mind was open to the thought of the shirt waist, but it was closed hard and fast against the idea of that particular store. At least the direct mental route to that store was closed. So the spirit had to lead me around by back alley brain-connections. But now the direct route is open.

The spirit always goes shopping with me, and nearly always the direct mental routes are open, so I have lots of fun shopping, never waste a lot of time at it, and I nearly always get just what I want, many times at bargain prices, though I almost never look at bargain ads in the papers. But many, many times have I gone into a store to buy a certain thing and found a big special sale on, of that very item.

65

Do you think these are very trivial things to be bothering the spirit about? I don't. The spirit is all-wise, all-powerful, everywhere present, *and its chief end and joy is to direct folks aright.*

The spirit is a sort of universal floor-walker to straighten out the snarls between supply and demand. in all departments of life. And I think it is a pretty heedless or foolish individual who won't consult it in every little dilemma.

And I notice that, in spite of this thought, I find myself ignoring the spirit—thinking I know of course where I'd better go for a shirt waist.

It seems hard to remember that Life's store is always growing and changing, so that we can always save time, money and needless meandering, by asking the spirit.

Herein lies the secret of all our little experiences when it looks as if our leading of the spirit was all wrong and our prayers, longing and desires all unanswered. The spirit never fails us. It is we who grow weary following the spirit; which must lead us to the desired goal by way of our own mental paths.

You see, it is a matter of cutting new streets in our mental domain, so it won't be necessary for the spirit to take us by such roundabout ways. It is a matter of clearing out our rocky prejudices so we'll not have to travel around them.

66

And here the spirit helps us again. As soon as the spirit succeeded in getting me around all my prejudices and into that store I wiped away the prejudice. So there is a straight mental street now where none existed before. The next time the spirit says "shirt waist," to me it can send me straight to D.'s if it wants to.

Yes, the spirit "moves in a mysterious way its wonders to perform." It looks mysterious to us until we are led back by the straight way. Then it is so simple, so easy, we can hardly believe the spirit would condescend to it!

Ah, but it does! Nothing is too small, or too great, for the spirit's attention—if we believe. When we don't believe we are to be pitied—and the spirit keeps discreetly mum.

I am the poet of the body and I am the poet of the soul.
The pleasures of heaven are with me and the pains of
*   hell are with me,*
The first I graft and increase upon myself, the latter I
*   translate into a new tongue.*

I am the poet of the woman the same as the man,
And I say it is as great to be a woman as to be a man.
And I say there is nothing greater than the mother of
*   men.*

I chant the chant of dilation or pride,
We have had ducking and deprecating about enough,
I show that size is only development.
*   —Walt Whitman.*

IX.

Spirit the Breath of Life.

"My healer teaches that I must depend alone upon Spirit; that breathing exercises, foods, sunshine and air must not be made the dependence for health. He says, 'Why, you can't help breathing.'"

That is tommyrot. Sunshine and air *are* spirit, and the plain truth of the matter is that if you don't use them all your "dependence on spirit" will avail simply nothing. Try living in a north room with the windows shut, and see.

You "can't help breathing," but your breathing avails nothing unless by it you take in good fresh live spirit in the way of pure air and sunshine. If we all lived under the sun and slept under the stars that healer's advice might be good enough. But we don't. We live in tight, dark rooms whence the spirit of life has fled, leaving only its cast off effluvia. We "can't help breathing," but what do we breathe? We breathe the dead air of close rooms.

Spirit is *LIFE, and we live by breathing it.* Spirit is in fresh air; fresh air is in spirit; fresh air and spirit are one. Dead air is air minus spirit, or life.

69

What good will it do you to say you depend upon
spirit when you don't; when you shut yourself away
from the spirit of life and breathe death?

Pure air and sunshine are spirit *specially prepared
for your use.* What good will it do you to pretend that
you depend upon spirit when you shut yourself into
rooms whence the spirit has flown?

If you live in close rooms you may "affirm" your dependence upon spirit until you are black in the face,
and you may be "treated" every hour of the day by this
healer and 10,000 more like him, and the result will be
only sickness and death.

I know in my heart and soul and mind that this is
true. And I have seen the truth of it demonstrated
by hundreds of cases of people who failed to get well on
"treatments" of any sort, and who afterward did get
well on sunshine, fresh air and full breathing, along
with mental treatment.

The Gospel of Fresh Air is more needed by human
beings than even the Gospel of New Thought. If we
understood and applied the Gospel of Fresh Air we
should think right without trying.

It is in gloomy, unaired corners that evil thoughts
breed—because the spirit of life is not present there in
such form that it can be appropriated by human beings.
They get therein the Breath of Death, and generate

70

thoughts to match—distorted thoughts of death and evil and despair.

Come into the sunshine and breathe the Breath of Life, which generates in you the New Thought of Life, Love, Wisdom, Truth, Health, Happiness, Success.

New Thought will not save you unless you live it, and a little observation and experimenting will prove to you that you *can't live it without breathing plenty of fresh air.*

If "all is spirit" why does this healer tell you that to regulate your breathing, exercise, food, etc., is to depend upon something outside spirit?

The fact of the matter is this: He fails to realize that all is spirit. He is still tangled up with good and evil, spirit and not-spirit, God and devil. He does not see spirit in everything and everything in spirit; so he puts the Keep-Off-the-Grass sign wherever he does not see spirit. This will not prevent his pointing you to the spirit where he does recognize it. None of us are wise enough as yet always to see God in all his works.

It is spirit which makes us breathe. When we shut ourselves away from the pure breath of life we shut away the power that makes us breathe.

And when we are too interested in doing indoor work the spirit finds it pretty hard work to make us breathe enough to keep us in good condition for growing. Close

71

rooms and sedentary work defeat the spirit's will to make us breathe.

So we, by working against the spirit, form a habit of breathing too little, thus robbing ourselves of the life, health, wisdom, power, joy which the spirit is trying to give us with every breath.

Now we find ourselves hampered by self-imposed habits which need breaking. So we set ourselves to work with the Spirit of Life. We throw open the window and let in the Spirit of Life.

We go out doors and revel in the Spirit of Sunshine.

We run and jump to make ourselves inbreathe the Spirit of Life.

Being too busy to spend hours every day outdoors we do stunts in our nightdresses to make us inbreathe more of the Spirit of Life.

And always, night and day, winter and summer, we take pains to leave our windows well open that the Spirit of Life be not shut away from us for one single moment.

We are learning to depend wholly upon the Spirit.

We used to remember the Spirit only on the Sabbath day; now we remember it every day and all day and all night—we remember to breathe it and eat it as well as think it.

And verily we are blessed.

X.

Affirmation and Wheels.

Mere repetition of "I Am Success" statements will avail little. One must think the thing he desires, and he must put his shoulder to the wheel. But the person who is full of the sense of failure and defeat is more apt than not to put his shoulder to the wrong side of the wheel. He is so discouraged and preoccupied and worried that he thinks it does n't matter much where he puts his shoulder, the thing won't budge anyway. So he goes stupidly along drudging away with his shoulder in the same old spot—the wrong spot.

But let that man make up his mind that there is a way to budge that wheel and he will find it; and you will see things move. That man will walk around that wagon a time or two, take in the lay of the land, pat his horses into willing humor, maybe back 'em up a bit, ring out a cheerful "Gid ap," and settle his shoulder to the right spot at the right moment—and away they go. Or another team will pass just at the right time to give him a lift out.

The man who believes himself equal to any emergency which arises will be strong mentally and physically. His mind will be alert, full of expedients. Instead of pushing like a blind mule at one spot until he drops in his tracks, he will use his gumption and find another way. He will conjure up a lever of some sort to budge that load. If he can't do it alone somebody else will come along in the nick o' time to give him the lift he needs. He believes he will work it somehow, and he does.

The "I Am a Failure" man never has anybody come along in the nick o' time. "Just my luck," he whines, and keeps on putting his shoulder to the wrong part of the wheel, or tugging hopelessly and half-heartedly, or—with inward rage that takes more energy than the tug—keeps on until he has to give it up for the time.

To affirm "I Am Success" will not pull the load out of the mire except as it awakes energy to intelligent effort. All affirmations and all going into the silence are useful in waking mental and physical energy to intelligent action.

All chronic failures are such because they believe in failure and opposition and "malicious animal magnetism" and general all-around the-world-is-against-me-ness. This belief in failure fills the individual with an affinity for undesirable things.

74

The infallible cure, the only cure, for failure, is belief in success, belief in one's own power to turn even defeat to good advantage. The man who "does n't know when he is beaten" will never be beaten. The "lunkhead" who "did n't know he was a lunkhead" went to the top, while the lunkhead who knew he was a lunkhead stayed at the lunkhead end of the class.

One of our big pork packers once tramped across the continent because he had n't money to pay his way. After he arrived at his destination he said he saw on his tramp hundreds of places where he could have started in without a cent and in time made piles of money—opportunities just crying to be developed. Only the thought of a bigger chance at the end of the route kept him from stopping in the very first town on his route!

But that boy had success in him and was on the alert for opportunities. He believed in himself and the world. The failure believes only in "bad luck" and his eye is out for "soft snaps," which he is certain he 'll never get a chance at. When a man is looking for trouble and defeat he finds them

"As a man thinketh in his heart so is he." That does not mean that a man may make a few affirmations of success, or profess new thought, and immediately become a success. The heart of man is the emotional center of

75

his habits or instinct, the center from which radiate his instincts, his habits, as the nerves radiate from the solar plexus.

Instincts are habit thoughts, heart thoughts. And every instinct came into being through conscious thought and effort. Follow your internal experiences while learning to play the piano, and you will gain a clear idea of how instinct comes into being. At first your fingers are stiff and every movement is a voluntary one, every movement has to be thought about, directed by thought. But gradually you acquire the habit of handling your fingers in a certain way. Gradually you cease to think at all about your finger movements; you "do it instinctively." In other words you have trained your heart, your subconscious mind, to do the thinking for you. Henceforth, instead of thinking consciously about your finger movements you think about them in your heart, that is, sub-consciously.

Psychologists say that not more than five per cent of our mental processes are conscious, the remaining ninety-five per cent being under the consciousness. This means that at least ninety-five per cent of our thoughts are habit thoughts, or "instinctive" thoughts. It is this instinctive part of us, this ninety-five per cent of us, that is referred to in the Bible as "the heart." Now if this "heart" of us carries at least

76

ninety-five per cent of our mentality you can easily see why a man is what he "thinketh in his heart." And you can see why a few affirmations of success, or even a good many of them, will not change the man sufficiently to make any great difference in his surroundings. And you can see why a mere intellectual conception of new thought is not enough to change him and his environment.

Man is a magnet, at least ninety-five per cent of which is habit mind. Therefore by far the greater part of his environment comes to him by its affinity to his ninety-five per cent habit or instinct mind, his under-conscious mind, of whose workings he is practically unconscious.

So it is no wonder he so often says, "I don't see why this undesired thing should come to me." He cannot see why it comes, because he is practically unconscious of that great ninety-five per cent of his thinking which draws them. He knows he does not consciously desire these unpleasant things and he can scarcely conceive the fact that he is conscious of only about five per cent of his thoughts and desires. And, too, he is loath to acknowledge that the greater part of himself has no more sense than to bring such things to him! He feels more complacent when he lays the blame at the door of "environment," or "wicked people," or "malicious

77

animal magnetism," or a "God who chastens whom he loveth," or a devil who got loose from God's leading strings and goes raging about to pester good folks.

Man is a magnet, and every line and dot and detail of his experiences come by his own attraction. "As a man thinketh in his heart so is he." The preponderance of attraction comes through the instinct self, the "heart."

And there is no use in trying to fight off, or run away from, the things which come to us. We only hurt ourselves by fighting. And to run away from the things we have attracted is to run into the arms of similar, or worse, conditions. We have to take ourselves along.

The only way to change conditions effectually is to change "the heart," the habit or instinct mind.

This can be done with more or less ease, according to the degree of setness of character and the degree of will and enthusiasm brought to bear.

The key to all change of character lies with that little five per cent conscious mind, which with all its littleness is a sure lever by which to move the ninety-five per cent ponderosity below it. For conscious thought is positive thought, dynamic; while subconscious thought is negative, receptive. That little five per cent mind has stronger compelling power than several times its bulk of subconscious mind, and *there is not an atom of*

78

*all that ninety-five per cent subconscious mind which
cannot be moved by that little five per cent mind which
lies at the top.*

The conscious self is the directing power. Just as
it directed your fingers to change their fixed habits, so
it can direct any change in other lines of mental or
bodily habit—by directing persistent, quietly insistent
practice on the desired lines. Insist upon right conscious thinking, and in due time you cannot fail to
have right subconscious thinking.

To think good, peace, love, self-command, self-faith,
success, long and faithfully enough will fill even the
most set "heart" with habits of good, peace, love, self-
command, self-faith, success. And *in proportion as the
heart becomes filled with such habits the environment
and experiences will change to match.*

How long will it take thus to transform you by the
renewing of your whole mind? All depends upon you.
If your practice is fitful and half-hearted it may take
another incarnation or two. If you go at it with a
steady will, cutting off all distractions which sap your
will and enthusiasm, practicing faithfully and diligently
at the new mental habits you may make the desired
change in, say, half a lifetime or less.

And if you can bring to your assistance a high spiritual exaltation and faith you can make the change in

79

almost no time at all. For spiritual exaltation and faith and enthusiasm will literally melt the hardest "heart" and permit a quick re-formation.

This is the secret of quick accomplishment in children; their hearts are clean and molten in the emotional fires of enthusiasm and faith, ready to receive deep and lasting impressions. By reason we grown-ups have cooled and even quenched the heart fires of faith and enthusiasm; so it takes time and repetition to reform us.

This is the secret of miracles. Religious enthusiasm and exaltation are akin to the fires of youth; they melt the heart to receive higher impressions.

The rationalist must receive his new impressions by painstaking hammering in. Repetition and time will do for him what religious or youthful enthusiasm does quickly for babes and fools.

No, affirmations will not do the work of "putting your shoulder to the wheel" when the load is stalled. But they will transform you, heart and consciousness, so that you will attract better horses as well as wheels, better roads, more friends to happen(?) around in the moment of need. And affirmations of the right sort will wake up your gumption so that you will not overload your horses or your personal energies to the point of needing a shoulder at the wheel.

Success is the natural result of intelligent direction of effort.

Affirmations of success, faith, wisdom, power, good, love, will wake your latent forces to more intelligent uses.

The more enthusiasm you can conjure into the affirmations the more quickly will you realize success.

April Rain.

It is n't raining rain to me,
It's raining daffodils;
In every dimpled drop I see
Wild flowers on the hills.
The clouds of gray engulf the day
And overwhelm the town—
It is n't raining rain to me,
It's raining roses down.

It is n't raining rain to me,
But fields of clover bloom,
Where any buccaneering bee
May find a bed and room.
A health unto the happy,
A fig for him who frets—
It is n't raining rain to me,
It's raining violets.

—Robert Loveman in Harper's.

XI.

Your Forces
and How to Manage Them.

You can overdo anything, even self-treatment. If you keep repeating affirmations to yourself your mental chattering interferes with the real healing.

It is not the conscious mind which heals you; it is the subconscious or soul mind and the super-conscious or Over-Soul mind.

Your soul's expression is guided and directed by your conscious mind. A mental affirmation is simply a word of direction to your soul mind. The soul hears your statements and then builds accordingly.

But what would happen if you called up your house-maids and told them over and over, just what you wanted done and just how to do it? If you spent all your time repeating your directions to them when would they get the work done? And would n't they get your directions mixed, too? Of course.

You don't do it that way, of course not; not if you are a wise housekeeper. You call up your maids and tell them quietly and kindly, and in as few words as possible, just what you want done. Then they go cheerfully away out of your presence and do their best to please you. If you later come across something which was not done right you call in a maid and repeat your directions, with perhaps a little further explanation. Then you go away again and trust her to do it aright this time.

What would happen if you tagged around after your maids and tried to watch and criticise and direct every little movement? Why, they would grow nervous and make foolish mistakes and you would all give up in despair.

And what would happen if you directed them to do a certain difficult piece of work and then came back five minutes later expecting to find it all done? Oh, you can't imagine yourself doing such foolish things!

Perhaps you don't with your maids, but evidently you do with your own self. Your objective, everyday consciousness is the mistress or master of your being. Psychologists say the objective mental activities are not more than one twentieth of all your mental activities. That means that the mistress mind has the equivalent of at least twenty maids under her direction. These "maids" belong to the subjective mind, or soul of you.

Then there is the great Over-Soul, of which your individual soul is but an atom; but an atom whose every demand is heard. That means that your little mistress mind not only has at her bidding the equivalent of at least twenty maids of the subconscious, but she has also at her call the equivalent of ten million billion other helpers of the infinite Over-Soul.

And all the mistress mind has to do is say the word. All these helpers fly to do her bidding.

Perhaps you think all these helpers don't fly to do your bidding. But they do. The only trouble with you is that you don't give your helpers time and chance to work out your desires. You keep repeating your directions over and over, and you keep trying to tag around after all your twenty or more housemaids to see if they are doing the things you want done. You watch them in your stomach and your liver and your lungs, always fretting for fear they are going wrong.

No wonder you get nervous and fidgety and strained all over; no wonder your "feelings" are no better than they were!

'Make your statements of health, happiness and success at certain regular intervals, say two or three times a day. Or make them at times when you can't get your mind off your conditions.

Make the statements plainly and positively. Then call your mind entirely away from the subject and give your soul and the Over-Soul a chance to work. Make light of your feelings and go get well interested in some good work.

Take it for granted that all your being, and all creation besides, is working out for you the things you desire. Rest easy and trust yourself.

Don't let your mind tag your feelings and symptoms; give it plenty of useful work and plenty of play and plenty of rest while your soul works things out for you as fast as it can. Just be as interested and happy as you can while the soul is working. *Jolly* yourself into having a good time.

Say the Word, and then be happy and do not allow yourself to doubt that the soul will do the work. This is the secret of quick healing. The nearer you can come to keeping your mind pleasantly occupied between the times when you give yourself special affirmations and treatments, the more quickly you will realize health of mind, body and environment as well as soul.

Thy faith in thy soul and the Over-Soul will have made thee whole.

The faithless mind is a terrible meddler and creator of discords; and the idle mind, the mind not directed to useful purposes, is always a faithless meddler. Moral: Get interested in some good work.

86

XII.

Duty and Love.

Though you work your fingers to the bone and have not love for your work it profits you next to nothing and your employer less than it ought to.

Duty work robs the doer of the joy of doing, which is the chief compensation for all work.

You imagine you do your work well from a sense of duty. You would do it better still if you loved it. If you loved it you would enjoy every bit of it, and you would glory in every little improvement you hit upon; and you would hit upon a lot because your soul would be playing through your fingers.

The soul of the duty doer is shut away from his work —he works with his fingers and his habit mind only. By the end of the week he is fagged out and his poor soul droops for lack of exercise; then perhaps he takes it to church for relief; and shuts it carefully away again before Monday morning.

And the worst of it is that so many people make a virtue of keeping their souls locked up six days out of seven. They parade duty as their mainspring. And

27

even when they do happen to let a little soul, a little love and joy into their work they won't acknowledge it. They stick to it that it is "duty" which impels them. When the soul does manage to get out of its shell and express itself in useful work the brain denies it the glory and happiness which belong to it. The worker resolutely shuts off the joy vibrations with that stern word "duty." He robs himself of the pleasure of his honest effort.

There are two ways of robbing one's self of the joy of work. One is by paralyzing joy with "duty"; the other is by scattering the mind and soul all over creation whilst the hands are doing something. In the former case the soul is shut away in idleness; in the latter it is wasted in riotous thinking.

The soul's power is emotion, that which flows from the silence within. The nature of emotion is motion.

To let emotion move through the body, out into intelligent effort, is joy and eternally welling life and strength and wisdom.

To let the mind wander while the hands work is to fritter your soul force away at the top of the head—the power which should move from the head down through the body and out into intelligent doing, is simply dissipated into thin air.

The wandering mind robs the body of vitality and

88

joy. It is the prodigal who wastes all your substance. The duty doer is a niggard. He lets some of his soul into his work, shutting the rest tight within. He puts his thought into his work, but he is stingy with his soul, his love. He works coldly, stolidly, conscientiously, reminding himself constantly that he is to "be good for nothing," as the wise mamma commanded the little boy who wanted a prize for being good.

Now everybody knows that cold contracts things. The cold duty doer shuts off his soul warmth and his body grows gaunt and pinched, his brain cells stiff, his thoughts angular. He shuts off the inspiration of love and joy and works like a machine, grinding out the same old things by the same old pattern.

The duty doer converts a real living, growing, loving being into a mere cold machine. It's a shame.

And the whole cause is the old fathers' tradition that duty is greater than love. I wonder where they got that notion?

The same spirit led them that leads us. That same spirit must have led them and us into duty doing.

Why? To gain self-control that we might have the greater joy. That is it! First there is the "natural," the animal way of doing things; just to follow impulse and gratify self at no matter what expense to others.

89

But somehow you are not very happy after you have done it.

Then there is the mental way of doing things, the "duty" way; when we cut off all the old "natural" impulses and teach ourselves to work stolidly, steadily in the "right" line. It takes about all our thought and effort to control ourselves in this mental way; it requires a firm unrelenting hand upon our impulses. But we were not happy when we didn't control our impulses, and we are at least at peace when we do. So we keep on crushing back the "natural" impulses and sticking sternly to duty. When we followed the old animal impulses to have things our way right or wrong, without regard to the other fellow, we were always lured on by the hope of joy; and when we got the thing desired, as we sometimes did, it was only to be disappointed. So we were full of unrest. Since we have chosen the ways of duty there are no joys to lure us, but rest accompanies us. In the old way we were always sure we were going to be happy; in the duty way we have ceased to expect happiness but we really have peace. And a peace in the heart, we have learned from sad experience, is worth two joys in the bush. We have been oft bitten and thus learned caution: so we keep on schooling ourselves to keep the peace and shut eyes and ears to promises of pleasure.

We have learned to f llow "conscience" instead of "natural impulse." Conscience is merely spiritual caution. The faculty called caution warns us from outward danger; it was created by many ages of race experience in getting its fingers burned and its shins kicked and its head broken. Conscience warns us from inner dangers; and is being created by many ages of human experience at stealing from the other fellow only to find its own heart robbed of peace and happiness. We tasted impulse and found it sweet at first and bitter, bitter at the last. Then we tasted duty and found its first pungency melt away to a clean sweetness such as we had never tasted before; a sweetness so pure and satisfying that it is no wonder we keep clinging to the duty doing which brought it.

When we lived from unchecked and unguided impulse only we were many times happy on the surface, when we happened to get the things asked for, but we were always restless and dissatisfied within This unrest is the voice of the universal spirit within, which is ever urging us to take our dominion over self and to direct our energies to higher and yet higher uses; it is the voice of life, which ever demands a high purpose for being and doing.

The spirit of the world which is moving us allows each a few years and many intervals of irresponsible

91

living. We have our childhood when the whole world smiles and flies to gratify every impulse; and when we are good children we have our little vacations and play happily with that sweet taste in our hearts. If we try to take too many play times the spirit in us is frowning and restless again, ever urging us to be up and doing that which will help the world spirit express the beauties it has in mind for us.

When we quit chasing pleasure and begin to live and do after the plan set in our hearts the world spirit whispers "Well done," to us. We find peace. We taste and see that it is good. Henceforth we work for the inner peace, not for the fleeting gratification of the outer senses.

As we follow duty peace deepens and widens. By and by we form the habit of duty and it grows easier and easier. We do what seems best because we have learned that to do otherwise ruffles our peace; and we have learned to love that peace beyond anything else life can hold for us.

Peace keeps on deepening and widening and growing more dynamic. At first it is a solemn calm, and a little deviation from duty ruffles and dissipates it. But by and by as we keep on doing our duty, through this solemn calm, growing ever deeper and broader, there wells the full diapason of a deep joy—very softly at first, with many diminuendos and silences; at unexpected moments it swells again; over little things the tide of life has brought us—things we loved, and thought we had given up forever when we chose duty as our guide. Fitfully at first the deep joy wells, fitfully and gently, but, oh, so full and sweet and satisfying; such tones as our souls never heard before. We wonder at the deep joy; and, oh, we begin to see that the world spirit was urging us on to duty only that we might find deeper joy than the old irresponsible life could yield us. By taking dominion over self, by using our energies for higher purposes, we have deepened our capacity for joy.

Now the harmony of deep joy begins to swell, and every touch of life but adds to the pæans of praise.

And the good things of life begin to come—houses, lands, fathers, mothers, brothers, a hundredfold more than ever before, bringing joy such as we never knew before. Oh, we thought we had given up the pleasures of life for its duties, and behold we find the pleasures added. We used to be fascinated and tossed about by life's pleasures; now we find them fascinated and obedient to us—oh, the power and glory and joy of it!

We gained dominion over ourselves and our environment through doing our duty. We gave up the shortsighted impulse will to follow the omniscient will which is working through us, and behold the things we once desired vainly are now ours to command and enjoy. No wonder we laud duty!

But duty is a schoolmaster whose work we do not need forever. When we have made its wisdom our own, we outgrow duty. Duty flowers in love.

The more resolution and persistence we put into duty doing the sooner we shall outgrow it.

The more pleasure we can get out of duty doing the faster we shall outgrow it. When the worker puts his soul into his duty, duty is swallowed up in love, and joy grows.

Many a duty worker cheats himself out of the joy which is his, and stunts the growth of his joy and himself, simply by denying that he works from anything but a sense of duty.

As long as our best efforts are called duty they answer to the call as cold, hard duty.

As soon as those same activities are called pleasures our soul joy, and love, are turned into them and they are transfigured.

The worker who calls his work duty shuts his soul back from his body and his work. The soul of you is love, and love has no affinity for duty; so as long as you insist upon working from a sense of duty you

94

shut in, shut away from your work, the sense of love.
You thus rob yourself of the joy of doing.

And this means that you rob yourself of the greater
share of your power and wisdom for doing.

Love is the essence of all wisdom, imagination and
inspiration, as well as power. To hold sternly to duty
is to shut out love, and with it the wisdom, inspiration
and imagination necessary to improve your work.
You are robbed of the joy of doing, and your work is
robbed of its highest beauty and usefulness.

Quit calling your duties by that name. Jolly yourself into doing your duty for love of it. Don't you
know how you can jolly a child into doing things?
Have n't you been jollied yourself until at last you
laughed and forgave and did the thing you had sternly
resolved not to do? Have n't you seen scores of your
friends jollied into doing things? Of course. All
nature responds to a smiling good-willed jolly.

And your soul, your love, will respond to the same
good-willed jollying. It will come out and smile on
your doings, and radiate soul-shine and joy and power
and inspiration through you, and down through your
fingers into your work, and out into your aura, and on
out to all the world.

Smile and come up higher than the duty class—the
joy class awaits you!

95

Express yourself.
Whatever you are, out with it!
We do not want a world of masqueraders;
Make yourself felt, make your real self felt.
Put your private stamp upon the future.
                                        —Ernest Crosby.

XIII.

Well Done.

"Natural disaster overtakes a man and he loses every cent. Possessing untold aversion to becoming a paid employee, he lives with friends, helping where able, and at the same time reaching out to grasp something by which to start again. Has an overwhelming desire to get money for home and marriage. This could be had in a very short time by successful speculation, if the unlimited Force is there as taught, for use on lines of desire. There is no wrong in the world. Is he then to command the powers for conscious use, go in faith and win; or shall he sit down and build, bit by bit, by uncongenial labor?"—M. T.

The man who possesses such "an untold aversion to becoming a paid employee" that he prefers to sponge a living off his friends rather than to earn it honestly, will never succeed even at speculation.

Such a man could not generate a desire strong enough to attract fortune even at a gambling table.

It takes *character* to generate a desire of the sort that moves things. It takes steadiness of purpose, positive determination.

And character, purpose, determination, are never found in the sponger.

If he had character he would choose any sort of honest work that would keep him in independence. His "un-

97

told aversion to becoming a paid employee" would be as nothing to his disgust for sponging a living, even temporarily.

Character is the outcome of an unconquerable self-respect and self-reliance. A man's character is that which distinguishes him from a jellyfish, which takes the shape of any environment that happens along. It is Something which keeps him upright on his own pins, no matter what happens.

Character is mental backbone and muscle, and is subject to the same laws of development and growth as other bone and muscle.

Bone and muscle and character do not grow by bread alone, but by use. Character grows by the use of self-reliance and self-respect, just as physical character grows by the use of muscles. Character becomes weak and flabby when self-reliance and self-respect are kept on the shelf of another man's pantry.

Character develops by exercise. How is it to exercise except by doing things? How is it to do things when somebody else does them for him?

The first thing a man of character, of self-respect and self-reliance would do under such circumstances as M. T. describes would be to overcome his "untold aversion" to anything which would help him to continue living in self-respect and self-reliance. In-

98

deed the only "untold aversion" held by a man of real character is the "untold aversion" to living off other people.

A person whose aversion to "becoming a paid employee" is greater than his aversion to idleness and sponging is a mere "mush of concession" to public opinion—he hates paid employment because he thinks his neighbors will "look down" upon him, and because he likes to look aristocratic and give orders rather than to be what he is and take what orders are necessary for the time being. Such a man cares for appearances above all things. He cares for the outside of things, as a jellyfish does. He seeks first an agreeable resting place, as the jellyfish does. And he will sacrifice the last vestige of self-respect, self-reliance, character, to that fetich, outside appearance. He thinks it looks better to live off his friends than to soil his hands to take care of himself.

But if he had a real character of his own, if he had mental backbone and muscle worthy the name, he simply could not crouch and cringe as a dependent, a beggar. He would have to get out and express himself in some sort of independent activity, or die.

For character is a deep-down life-urge which will push to expression through any conditions. It simply cannot continue to sit supinely by another man's fireside, or wait by the wayside with cap extended to catch stray pennies from the passers-by.

Character must act, or degenerate.

Character must ex-press, or ex-pire.

Character is to the individual what the channel is to the river. Take away the banks which confine the stream and direct it and the water gushes out in an endless sloppy marsh.

The inner character of a man confines and directs the life force, the desire force; the stronger the character the deeper and broader the stream of desire, or life; and the more positively the man will express himself in independent, self-respecting activity. The stronger the character the greater will be the man's "untold aversion" to depending upon anybody but himself. And so deep and strong are his desires as they flow through the clear-cut channels of character, that they force new channels through any circumstances. Such a man's desires flow deep and strong enough to carry things his way.

But the man without a strong character is a mere sloppy marsh of sentimentality. He is incapable of anything more than "overwhelming desires"—his desire stream, having no strong banks, simply overwhelms the whole surface of things, with no depth by which to sweep its way through environment. His desire energy

100

spreads out and wastes itself in mere shallow longings, unworthy the name of desire. So the man welters in his own swamp of sensibility, and gets nowhere.

Herein lies the reason that M. T.'s man will not find success at the gaming table, nor anywhere else, except by "building bit by bit" a character strong enough to find its way to the good things he wants.

The first step toward success is to decide that it is yours, and that all creation is ready to help you manifest it.

The next step is to work with the world, taking hold anywhere that the world will let you, in full confidence that the world will promote you as fast as you prove your fitness for promotion.

To prove your fitness for promotion necessitates doing your best with any job the world gives you, and at the same time using your spare time and thought in fitting yourself for a better one.

To do one of these things is not enough. The man who does his work exceptionally well will be kept at that same kind of work until crack o' doom unless he shows aptitude for doing more valuable work. The world is always looking eagerly for men who can fill the more difficult positions. It is always trying to tempt people into higher, better paying positions; and the man who is faithful and efficient in one place, and

101

evinces the slightest capacity for higher work, is always the first man to get a chance of promotion.

The man who thinks he is "kept down" is right; but he is kept down by himself alone. Either he is slack, inefficient, uninterested, gumptionless in his present work; or he is not fitting himself for something better.

Abe Lincoln split rails all day. He split them with vim and intelligence. But at night he studied books by the light of a pine knot. All the way along from rail splitting to the presidency, Abe found some time out of business hours to inform himself on lines beyond his work.

The main difference between Abe Lincoln and Abe Johnson lies in the way they spend their after-business hours. Abe Johnson, too, works with vim and intelligence. And he never had to split rails for a living. He is an A1 bookkeeper. Been in the same store, with almost the same salary, for twenty-five years. And almost every noon and every evening for twenty-five years he has sat on a sugar keg in the store and discussed politics and economics. And very often he has grumbled to his cronies about his lack of a chance to rise in the world.

Down here in a Massachusetts town, they have been having labor troubles for a long time. The cotton mill owners say the bottom has dropped out of the plain

102

cotton cloth trade and they simply must reduce wages or close down. There is small demand for the sort of plain cotton goods manufactured in these mills. The mill hands say they can't live on any smaller wages and they won't, so there. So one strike follows another, or a lockout. For months at a time the mills lie idle while owners and workers deadlock.

Some one suggested that the mills begin to make the sort of new fancy weaves of cotton cloth for which there is increasing demand. But the weavers refused to learn the new weaves. They said they knew how to do the plain weaving and it "would n't pay them" to learn the new kind of weaving on the old wages, which are paid according to the amount of work done. And many of them said anyway they were too old to make such changes now.

So these faithful and efficient weavers go on fighting and striking and reviling "fate" rather than fit themselves for new work which would in the end pay better than the old.

Poor shortsighted weavers.

Poor shortsighted cousins to the weavers. Poor shortsighted and disappointed Abe Johnson.

* * * * * * *

What do you suppose life makes us begin at the bottom for, and "build bit by bit"? For the sole purpose of building character; building good, strong channels for desire to run in; channels so deep and full that the desire-stream will be strong enough to accomplish for the individual the thing he wants.

And how are we to know we are building the right kind of character? By the sense of inner satisfaction which witnesses every well done deed.

That is where self-respect and self-reliance come in. Even a baby feels the "Well done" of its soul when it succeeds in doing something for itself. A child prizes this inner self-satisfaction, self-respect, above all things else. Watch the happy look on a child's face when it has succeeded in doing something for itself.

Only foolish grown-ups value anything on earth above this inner satisfaction. Only grown-ups will let other folks do for them what they can do for themselves. Only grown-ups will quench themselves for the sake of appearances. Some grown-ups.

To know thyself is to know that the best thing in heaven or earth, the best guide in heaven or earth, is the inner sense of "Well done," the sense of self-respect which comes from doing things instead of letting them be done for you.

As long as the innermost self approves your doings you are building character. And what shall it profit you if you gain the whole world and lose the "Well done" of your soul? Nothing! Less than nothing! For in all creation or uncreation there is but one real satisfaction, one real happiness, and that is self-satisfaction, self-respect.

Self-respect springs only from well-doing. It is "Well done," thy soul says to thee, that gives thee joy.

What matter what Tom, Dick, and Harry and Madame Grundy say? Be still and hear thyself.

Eye hath not seen nor ear heard the glory and satisfaction which await him who listens to himself.

"Well done, good and faithful servant; enter thou into the joy of thy Lord"—which is thy innermost self.

The Barred Door.

One night upon mine ancient enemy
  I closed my door,
And lo! that night came Love in search of me—
  Love I had hungered for—
And finding my door closed went on his way
  And came no more.
Pray you take counsel of this penitent
  And learn thereof:
Set your door wide whatever guests be sent
  Your graciousness to prove.
Better to let in many enemies
  Than bar out Love.
          —Theodosia Garrison in Harper's Bazar.

106

XIV.

What Has He Done?

We were talking about new thought and the increased efficiency it gives to people. Evidently he did not think very highly of the practical side of new thought. It is all very well to help people to bear their troubles, he said, but it does not get rid of the troubles.

And I said I thought if it never did anything more than help people to endure things, it at least helps more than anything else ever did.

But I assured him that new thought rightly applied does change conditions, and I cited my own experience in proof. Then I called his attention to other people, prominent in the new thought, whose conditions and health have been changed for good. One of the names mentioned was that of a successful lawyer well known to us both. "Well," queried he, "what has he done that is so wonderful? Others have done as great or greater things, who never heard of new thought."

Of course. The principles of new thought are the principles of life itself, and in all climes and times there have been people who, consciously or unconsciously, lived according to principle and thereby manifested health (which means wholeness) of mind, body and environment.

Wisdom's ways are always ways of pleasantness and all her paths are peace.

And wisdom is as omnipresent as the ethers, to be used by him who inspires it—by him who desires it above all else.

Every pleasant thing and thought in this world comes by mental breathing of wisdom. And every soul that ever lived has lived by breathing wisdom.

In proportion to his inbreathing of wisdom has been the pleasantness of his ways and the peace of his path.

And his ups and downs have come from the fact that he inspires wisdom in spots only. He keeps on mentally breathing, of course; but he does n't always breathe wisdom. He is like a man who breathes pure outdoor air awhile, and then goes into a close room, or down in a mine, and breathes poison gases.

As physical health depends upon the quantity of pure air inspired, so physical and mental and environmental health depends upon the amount of pure wisdom inspired.

And nobody will deny that most of us inspire a large proportion of poison gas of the mental kind, instead of pure wisdom. We breathe over other people's thoughts after them, just as we breathe over the air after them. This breathed-over thought destroys our physical, mental and environmental health. We need to get out in God's open and breathe new thought, or we shall asphyxiate.

Old thought is division, dissension, separateness, competition.

New thought is the great open of principles, oneness, harmony, God, good, freedom, peace, love.

New thought is from ages to ages everlasting. Those who inspire it, inbreathe it, are the whole and strong ones, whether they breathe it consciously or unconsciously.

By teachings of new thought the world is learning to do consciously, intelligently, what a few have done here and there through all the ages. And need we be reminded of the advantages of knowing how and why we do things?

"What has he done that is so wonderful?" The lawyer we spoke of is not what the world calls "great" in any line. He has not built up a Standard Oil "system," nor torn one down. He is not a Roosevelt or a Togo, or a Napoleon, nor even an Elbert Hubbard. His desires and ambitions have run in other lines. He is not "built that way." He "has n't it in him" to be a Rockefeller, and he is glad of it.

109

Why then should he be compared with Napoleon or Rockefeller? Do we measure roses and violets and daffodils and chrysanthemums by the same standards? Is the violet inconsequential because it sheds its sweetness in a shady corner instead of flinging it in midday from the top of a sunflower stalk? No. We measure violets by other violets, not by sunflowers or hollyhocks or peonies.

And men are more diverse than flowers. Every man has his own individuality, his own soul specifications to develop by. Every man comes as the flower of a peculiar ancestry, like no other man's ancestry. To judge one man by another is as foolish as to judge a violet by a sunflower.

This lawyer we spoke of stands in a class by himself. He has not achieved what Rockefeller has, but he has achieved something which satisfies himself better than the doings of a dozen Standard Oil magnates could.

And what is success but self-satisfaction?

To succeed is to accomplish what one sets out to do.

A growing success is a matter of growing ideals and a succession of successes.

Our lawyer is satisfied with new thought and its efficacy in his case. By its use he has accomplished a succession of things he wanted to do. He has literally made himself over, and his environment, too. And he has evolved new ideals and developed new energies which show him a joy-full eternity ahead.

He is satisfied with the new thought as a working principle.

He goes on working by it, growing daily in wisdom and knowledge, daily growing greater graces of character, mind, body and environment.

It is the man who does not live new thought teachings who misjudges them by the outward appearances of other men's lives.

Nothing before, nothing behind;
  The Steps of faith
Fall on the seeming void, and find
  The Rock beneath.
                    —Whittier.

XV.

Will and Wills.

In a copy of an old magazine is an article entitled, "What New Thought Women Say of the Will, by an Old Thought Woman," who fails to sign her name. This article is about as cross-eyed as anything I have read recently. It amuses me. And yet it touches a responsive chord of stored memories, and I sympathize. That is, I am enabled for the moment to re-enter the same-pathy or condition this woman describes. Every step she has passed through I, too, have experienced.

But I have passed through it all and emerged upon the spiral above, where I am enabled to understand the phenomena of wills in relation to each other, and in relation to the whole.

Briefly stated, "The Old Thought Woman's" idea is, "The will is a part of that delusive mortal mind. It is the executor of the world, the flesh and the Devil. 'God's will' is a fiction." "Devil" with a capital D, mind you. Then she goes on to tell how willful she used to be; she dominated her relatives, friends and enemies alike, and even the cats and dogs. "There was

113

scarcely no way in which will can dominate that I did not work to its limits," she says; "I intended to marry without declaring my views, get the property and support, but refuse all sensuality," because she was "adamant against child-bearing."

Decidedly a disagreeable person, I should say. I don't wonder that she was "cordially hated by those whom she hypnotized and outwitted"; I don't wonder "pain, anguish, hatred, suffering, disappointment followed in the wake of every triumph." Do you?

Then she grew sick of it all and "gave up all will." "In a complete loss of will, self-will, God's will, all kinds of will, there is a miraculous condition of affairs," she says. Then she goes on to preach Christ's teaching of non-resistance.

Every positive character, and probably every negative one, too, passes sometime through an experience identical with this woman's. The more pronounced the character the more definite is the change from self-will to self-abnegation. A negative character will *hang on* eternally to his self-will, and the *giving up* of his will causes him all the anguish this woman experienced as a result of *using* her will.

Now without pointing out to you the mistakes of this writer let me give you my statement of will, its nature and uses; after which I think you will see the Old Thought Woman's understanding needs to grow a bit.

Will is the motive, electric force of the universe; the only force there is.

Will is the energy which forms worlds and swings them in space; which dissolves all forms and creates anew.

Will is attraction and gravitation.

Will is love, and will is hate.

Will is the passion, the active force, of the One.

Will is omnipresent and omnipotent.

Without will there could be only stagnation, death, annihilation.

But there is Will; and there are wills; there is all-pervading, all-evolving Will, and there are countless little tossing, warring wills. There is one great ocean, and there are countless little, tossing wavelets, each taken up with its own aims to rise above its neighbors.

On the unseen side Will is one, the only One. On the seen side there are only wills, beginning and ending within the personal circle.

Will is the executive of omniscience.

Will is the executive of universal, all-evolving Wisdom. "Will of God" is no fiction; it is the one immutable, inexorable FACT which personal wills ceaselessly and uselessly toss themselves against, to their undoing *and the increase of knowledge.*

All-Wisdom and All-Will are the one great ocean,

115

from which personal wisdom and will are tossed, and to which all return.

Will and Wisdom are all there is in the universe; they are one and inseparable. Water is correctly formulated as W^2W, instead of H^2O; and every atom in the universe, seen or unseen, is simply Will in definite and varying proportion to Wisdom. The less Wisdom in the mixture the more foolishly will the Will be exercised.

Will is used commonly as a name for volition exercised by the conscious 5 per cent mind. The individual reasons from his own narrow view and sets his will to execute his finite judgments. For the time he sets his judgment up as infallible, grits his teeth, clinches his fists and drives through;—until he comes slam up against Universal Will. It is as if one of your hands set up a judgment of its own and attempted to force the other hand to move after his pattern. Your right hand sees and judges for a right hand, but not for a left hand.

Just so with this Old Thought Woman; she set up her judgment and attempted to bring relatives, friends, enemies, animals, under subjection.

Under subjection to what?—her will? *No—under subjection to her judgments.* Her will was simply the executive—the sheriff's posse. Having a strong will she had her way in many cases, where a less determined

116

individual would have held just as severe judgments without having the will to execute them.

Was her will "evil," a "delusion"? No. But her wisdom was a minus, a *personal*, quantity and her will thereby misdirected.

I am a very strong willed woman and I glory in it. But the time was when I made all kinds of a chump of myself by setting up my judgment for other people's guidance, and sending my will to execute my judgments, willy nilly on the other fellow's part. My *will* was first class; likewise my intention; but my judgment was exceedingly narrow and crude. I got into all kinds of hot water, just as this Old Thought Woman did; and finally I could n't stand it any longer.

I "went to the Lord." I prayed and agonized and humbled myself—as I needed to. The trouble with me was that I had not learned yet that *my* judgments were not the best on earth and *my* will the only executive. All these failures on my part made me look at last for higher judgments and mightier will.

Among men I could not find them. Not a writer or lecturer or friend but showed me plainly that his judgments were as wry and his will as circumscribed as my own. So I turned to the unseen and unbelieved-in, but greatly needed and longed for God. I "gave up my will"—I said, "Not my will but thine be done."

It was hard to do, but being a strong willed woman I did it and did it well. I lived daily with Jesus in that sublime "Sermon on the Mount."

Of course "I found peace." Having laid aside all personal aims and ambitions and given up all efforts to make myself or the world better, I found peace.

An Indian lying full length in his canoe, which is floating softly and surely down the broad Columbia toward the ocean, is an emblem of peace.

The individual who wakes up at last to the fact that what he has been tearing himself in tatters trying to accomplish *is already being* accomplished by a broad river of Will of which his own will is but a wavelet, finds himself incarnating peace.

"He that loseth his life shall find it." *He that loseth his will shall find it*—for the first time.

I thought I was giving up my will, when it was only my judgments I gave up. And I gained in return *the entire will of the universe.* I changed my point of view —that was all. I had been seeing countless myriads of striving, tortured individuals, each warring in chaos to bring order according to his judgments.

Now I saw God as the animating *soul and will and wisdom* working in and through and by these striving ones.

From a formless wavelet striving to *get up,* I became

the Indian, resting, realizing the mighty Will underneath me that carried me unerringly in the right direction *even when I did nothing.*

I rested and let the All-Will carry me *and everybody else.* At times it seemed that I *must* spring up and *make* this one or that one go right or do right. But I *used my will on myself* and kept hands off. I could not *see* that the All-Will was bringing this out right; but *I* had made such a miserable failure when *I* was running things that in sheer despair I *determined* to resist nothing, compel nobody, but just *trust* that the All-Will would bring things out right.

I kept saying to myself, "Hands off—hands off—loose him and let the All-Will run him," until I really learned to *let* the All-Will do it.

Of course I thought, just as this Old Thought Woman does, that *I* was exercising no will at all. But I was, and she is doing it, too. The only difference between the use of my will before and after this self-abnegation was this: After I "gave up my will" I `had the All-Will on my side for the first time,* and so easy did it seem to be to let the All-Will do everything, that I did not realize that the All-Will *worked through and by my personal will.* It was as if I had been trying desperately to lift something too heavy for me, and suddenly my efforts were reinforced to such an extent that it was

119

easy. Or, as if I had been trying hard to shove open what seemed a door when along came one who showed me where the real door was and how to open it easily.

I had been using all my will to make myself and others "good" and suddenly I found the All-Will reinforcing my little will—as if a mighty power had been switched on to my circuit.

This was not really what happened, you know. It was this: My little will had been striving *against* other little wills—as if one finger strove to curtail the action of another finger. At last, in desperation and without at the time understanding what I did—I let go my little attempt; and immediately I began to sense the All-Will working through my will for the accomplishment of larger purposes I had not before dreamed of.

It was hard to strive against other wills—hard; and the outcome uncertain, and fraught with suffering and disappointment. But it was *easy* to let the All-Will *back* my will—so easy I failed for some time to realize I was using any will.

Like Solomon I asked for wisdom, for understanding. As it came to me I saw that whenever the All-Will backed my will and made action easy I was on the right track; whenever I felt a sensation of pulling against some other will I was on the wrong track and must let go and rest. Many times the thing I could not at one time do without that *pulling against* feeling, at another time I could do easily with that sense that the All-Will backed me. Sometimes the All-Will backed me in doing what some other person opposed, and yet I was not backed when *I* did the opposing.

At first all this seemed like the capricious "leadings" of a "spirit." But at last I began to see a principle in it.

I found the Law of Individuality. I found that when I willed to do anything which *I* desired, the All-Will backed me, *unless* I foolishly desired to *curtail what some other body desired to do—not* what some other body desired *me* to do, but what he desired to do *without interference with me.* Do you see the point? For instance, I desired to teach and heal; another desired me to cook and sew; *and the spirit backed me.* I serenely taught and healed. That other fumed and fretted, and yet, all serene, I *knew* the All-Will backed *me*. But that other smoked; I considered smoking wasteful and detrimental; and every time I expressed my opinions on the subject I felt that the All-Will was *not* backing me. This one had a *right* to smoke, because he was not thereby interfering with the free action of another. But when he tried to put me back in the kitchen he had to use his *personal* will unbacked by the All-Will; because the All-Will was backing *my* will to get *out* of the kitchen. On the other hand, the

121

All-Will backed *his* will to smoke; therefore when I tried to interfere I opposed not only his will but the All-Will as well.

Now that is just what gives us all so many hard knocks in the world, dearie. We fail to respect the other fellow's rights, and in so doing we run against not only his personal will but the All-Will into the bargain. No wonder we get some horrible bumps.

When you exercise your will against another's freedom of action you shut yourself off from your source of will supply, the All-Will. This is why you clinch your fists, grit your teeth and contract your lungs and muscles. You are shut off from the source of will supply, and you *contract* in order to *force your will power against another*. Then you are exhausted, and have accomplished nothing. For if you succeed in "making him be good" this time he hates you for it. And he will break out with more force at the next opportunity—*because the All-Will is backing him* even in the actions *you* judge as "bad." Remember, the All-Will backs *every* personal will except when the personal will interferes with the free *action* (not interference) of another will.

Then, when you attempt interfering with the free action of another you force out your will upon him, just as you force out the breath from your lungs. Then

122

you have to "catch your breath" and your will again. It takes time to fill yourself again with will, and whilst you are doing it you suffer all those horrible sensations of remorse and weakness and disgust that come over one after one of these tussles with another will. You have all these feelings whether or not you succeed in downing the other fellow. Oh, it does n't *pay,* dearie. It does n't pay to use your will except when you can feel the All-Will backing you.

What new thought people refer to as "cultivating the will" is simply cultivating acquaintance with and consciousness of the All-Will. It is simply *recognition* of will; recognition of the ceaseless, underlying urge of the universe which is working within and through the individual to express more and more of beauty and wisdom and good.

To use the little, personal will apart from the All-Will one must *contract* and thus *force out* his will upon other people and things.

To use the All-Will one must first know he is right, then *relax* and *let* will flow through him to accomplish according to his word or desire.

In using the little, personal will one recognizes himself a member of a multi-verse—a being separate and apart from all other beings.

In order to use the All-Will one must first have

123

learned his relation to it and to all other persons and things; he must have recognized the uni-verse, and himself and others as orderly, useful members of the universe.

Only as he recognizes Oneness is it possible for him to resign the exercise of the small, personal will and *let* the All-Will accomplish through himself and through every other man.

He that loseth his will shall find it one with All-Will.

And after all it is not his will he has lost, *but his beliefs about it and its use.* He has come up higher and caught a glimpse of the unity of things. He has hitched his wagon to omnipotence and behold all things are done according to his word.

The All-Will backs the individual in *anything* good, bad or indifferent, which he wills to do; just so long as the individual does not interfere with other individuals. So you see, in any effort you may make toward self-development you have All-Will working with and through you. And if you will attend strictly to business nothing on earth or in hell can stem the tide of your will, and so defeat you.

> "There is no chance, no destiny, no fate,
> Can circumvent or hinder or control,
> The firm resolve of a determined soul."

XVI.

Concerning Vibrations.

Vibration is Life. Vibration is motion. All motion is vibration. All motion is Life. You expand your chest with an inhalation of air; you contract your muscles and exhale. This is vibration. Your heart "beats." This, too, is vibration.

Every tiny cell in your body is "beating," or vibrating, just as your heart and lungs do. When your chest expands you take in fresh air, which goes not only into your lungs, but into all parts of your body. The air blows like a fresh breeze around the countless millions of cells which go to make up your body. These little cells in their turn expand and take in the air. Then the cells contract and force out the air, and your lungs, too, contract, and force the air clear out of your body.

Now this air which is thus vibrated through your body serves to clean it. The decaying particles of your body cells are thrown off and carried out in the streams of air which are vibrated through your body. If it were not for this vibration of your body, which keeps

125

the air flowing through, your body would soon become clogged with dead matter.

The nerves and arteries in your body are constantly contracting and expanding, contracting and expanding, to move along the blood, which carries food. supply to the cells and bears away their sewage in just the same way that the air is carried to and from the cells.

It is by constantly vibrating—contracting and expanding—that your stomach and bowels digest food.

It is by vibration of the cells of tree and plant that the sap flows through and feeds the tree.

Even a stone is composed of tiny cells which breathe, just as the cells of your body, and just as your body as a whole does.

Every individual, be it cell, plant, animal or man, lives by vibrating; by expanding and contracting to take in the new and force out the old matter. Every mind, too, lives by vibrating—by alternately expanding to receive new ideas and contracting to get rid of the old.

Then there is another sort of vibration by which one individual communicates with another. Imagine to yourself that the ether is made up of infinitely small elastic balls. If you strike any one of those tiny balls it will strike those next to it and rebound, and those hit will strike the next, and so on the blow will travel from one tiny ball to the next, clear to the edge of creation—if you can imagine such a place. The blow you strike sets all the little elastic balls to vibrating, or moving back and forth.

Now if I stand away out in space and I feel the little elastic balls vibrate against me I know it means Something. By experience I learn what each kind of movement means. If you clap your hands together the vibrations of those tiny elastic balls strike my ear and I say, "I hear some one clapping hands." If I face your way the vibrations strike my eyes and I say, "I see some one clapping hands." In any case your motion caused the ether to vibrate and I felt the vibrations. If I had no ears or eyes I could not feel the vibrations, but they would be there just the same.

Every movement made sets the ether to vibrating to its particular pitch; and wherever there are eyes or ears the vibrations are recorded. When you talk it sets the ether going just the same whether there are ears to hear or not.

And when you keep perfectly quiet and think you set the ether going, too. Your brain sets vibrations going, just as your tongue does. There are people who can hear thoughts, just as you hear another's speech. In

127

due time we shall all hear thoughts—we are all growing mental ears.

Thoughts are higher vibrations than spoken words; and they "carry" farther. You know a deep, growly bass voice makes a great noise when you are close to it, but a shrill treble call can be heard much farther than the growly bass. The high voice makes short, sharp, far-reaching vibrations. Now thoughts make infinitely shorter, sharper and farther-reaching vibrations than the voice can; and thought vibrations carry farther and far more quickly.

And wherever there is another thinker ready to hear, the thoughts are recorded.

Many times we hear the thoughts of other people and mistake them for our own; for everybody has at least a little mental hearing.

When you speak clearly and distinctly your voice carries much farther than if you speak hurriedly and carelessly; and other people can more readily understand what you say. If you mumble your thoughts or your words the etheric vibrations carry mumbled meanings.

As people learn to think distinctly their thoughts carry farther and find more listeners. In course of time and with due practice, we shall easily think so that people on the other side of the earth can hear us. Not only that, but we shall think so clearly and high that the inhabitants of Mars and Venus and the sun, too, shall easily hear us.

I should n't wonder if what we call sun rays are really the thought vibrations of the sun's inhabitants. What if we receive and respond to their thoughts and think them our own!

According to the original Christian teaching (as I understand it), all undesirable conditions and circumstances are constituted by illusions that are held by ignorant, immature minds, and that project on to the bodily or material plane what may be compared to shadows. "If thine eye be single"—that is, if thy view be true, if thy understanding of life be sound,—"thy whole body shall be full of light. But if thine eye be evil, thy whole body shall be full of darkness." Undesirable experiences are the darkness wherein a person walks and works and stumbles about, whose notion of the universe, instead of shedding light on the meaning of life, casts on it a shadow. They are the effects produced on the field of our senses, by mistaken thought on the main issues of life, by a misunderstanding of life, by believing, and therefore practicing, a lie. The stuff they are woven of is something like the unsubstantial kind of stuff that makes up nightmares. They are the sort of thing from which Truth, thoroughly known, can set people free.

—J. Bruce Wallace.

XVII.

The I Was and the I Am.

Some one has said that "an honest man is the noblest work of God." Ten thousand thousand others have repeated his little speech—with a solemn wag of the head and sidewise squinting which conveyed the opinion that God is chary of his noble works.

Then there came another man who paraphrased that. "An honest God is the noblest work of man," he said. And a thousand or so of us wondered why we had n't thought to say that! Why, of course. And the other thousands of thousands lifted up their hands and cried, "Blasphemy—stone him, stone him—put him out of the church, where the bogies 'll get him!" They put him out. But the bogies have n't got him. And many of the thousands are taking up his cry—"An honest God is the noblest work of man."

Why not? An honest God is of greater value than many honest men, is he not? God is the creator of man; unless God is himself honest his honest man is but an accident, instead of an image and likeness of himself.

131

But, according to the paraphraser, man creates his God. Well, that is a paraphrase only, and true only in a sense.

God is. Man's creation of God is simply his mental concept of God; it is God as he sees him, or it, from his viewpoint. An honest God is the concept of a man whose soul recognizes honesty and loves it. A God of power is the mental creation of him whose soul recognizes and loves power. A God of love is the mental creation of him who recognizes and loves love. A God of vengeance is the mental concept of him who loves vengeance.

Perhaps you think your mental concept of God is not so very important, since it is all in your mind and the real God is what he is regardless of your idea of him. But it matters vitally to you. It is not God as he really is, that is creating you; but God as he appears to you. Your concept of God is creating you in its own image and likeness. If you think of God as a great man on a throne, with a long white beard and an eye-for-an-eye-and-a-tooth-for-a-tooth expression, you may depend upon being made over into a sour-visaged decrepit old man who will want to die and get away from it all.

If you think of God as a God of power, love, wisdom, beneficence, you will aim to be perfect as he is perfect.

132

If you happen to be one of the fools who has said in his heart there is no God, your life will be a crazy patchwork and your end that of the stoic who defies earth to do its worst by him; which it probably will, being a willing earth and ready to give each according to his demands.

You are being created in the image and likeness of the Lord your God, the God enthroned in your heart. What kind of a God is in your heart? Is he small and revengeful and capricious, a sort of policeman to tell your troubles to, to receive consolation from, and by whom to send punishment to your enemies?

Or is your God the Principle and Substance behind all creation, the power, wisdom, love, of all creation, a God who loves all, is just to all, generous to all, favors none?

But no matter how lofty a God you carry in your heart he will do you little good unless he is an I Am God.

Most men's Gods are I Was Gods. They believe God did wonderful things for the children of Israel; that he performed great miracles for the apostles and disciples of Jesus; but to this age they think of him as merely the I Was God, who stands aloof and lets man run things—man and the devil, or "malicious animal magnetism."

133

Believers in the I Was God are also great sticklers for the I Shall Be God, who is coming again to judge the wicked and set up his kingdom on earth. And these believers in the I Shall Be God think that their only business in life is to wait around until the great I Shall Be makes his appearance.

People who worship the I Was and the I Shall Be are never demonstrators. Between admiration of the I Was and anticipation of the I Shall Be they fall to the ground and—wait for the I Shall Be in themselves and others.

Only the I Am God does things. I Am love impels you to love now. I Am wisdom inspires you to act upon your ideas. I Am power performs miracles, not yesterday or to-morrow, but now. I Am God is the God who works to-day, in you and in me. His ways are not the ways of the I Was God, nor of the I Shall Be God; they are the ways of the I Am—new, different, the ways of to-day, not of yesterday or to-morrow.

I know a dear woman who worships the I Was and the I Shall Be. She entertained Schlatter the healer, and was firmly convinced that he was a literal reincarnation of Jesus Christ. She took Schlatter's word for it. She also accepted his excuses for not immediately setting up a literal kingdom here on earth, as described in the book of Revelations. He told her he had other work to do just now, that he was going away, but would soon return and establish a literal kingdom. She swallowed it all—without a single chew. Schlatter went away, and later a body was found in the mountains which was said to be his.

Since Schlatter's disappearance, some years ago, this lady has spent her time in writing about him and looking for his return. The I Was and the I Shall Be absorb her entire spiritual attention.

In the meantime she lives in a small mining town where in the life surging about her she sees no God. Not long ago she wrote me to help her speak the Word of freedom for a man on trial for his life. She said he was absolutely innocent and that a "terrible conspiracy" existed against him. The man was condemned to die, still protesting, not innocence but self-defense. It was a case of mix-up with two men and a woman, followed by a drunken brawl and the usual plea of "did n't mean to."

This lady's sympathies were all with the man, and her letters to me were pitiful. Her heart was wrung with agony for him and his bereaved wife, and convulsed with horror and impotent rage at the "wickedness" of the "wretches who falsely swore away his life." The way "evil" triumphed over justice was awful, she said, and she knew when Schlatter returned justice would be done and the wicked wretches annihilated—or words to that effect.

You see, she has no conception of an I Am God, who rules now. She sits in judgment on men's acts and prays to Schlatter to come back and set things right. She remembers that the I Was put 10,000 to flight with Gideon's three hundred pitchers and candles—simply sneaked up and scared them into a panic. She knows the I Was hardened the heart of Pharaoh to lie repeatedly to the Israelites. She knows the devil had to ask permission of God before he tempted Job. She knows God said "I make peace and I create evil," and that "The Lord hath made all things himself; yea, even the wicked for the day of evil." She knows that "Whatsoever the Lord pleased that did he in heaven, and in earth, in the seas, and all the deep places." She knows all these things of the Great I Was. But that the I Am works now in the hearts of men; that God now hardens one heart to perjury and another to truth, one to murder and another to lay down his life that his friend may live;—that God now works in these apparently antagonistic ways and thereby works out perfect justice, wisdom, love, has never entered her mind. She cannot imagine that no man meets any form of death until he himself has ripened for that particular form of death. She has read that eighteenth chapter of Ezekiel,·

136

where God explains that every man dies for his own sins, not for the false swearings of another. But the great I Was said that, and the I Shall Be says it; but the I Am is absent—so she thinks.

Somewhere in the Old Testament—in Psalms, I think—the statement is made that those who die are "taken away from the evil to come." I opine that this is literally and unvaryingly true, that death never comes except as the dying one needed relief from worse things than death, things which lay straight ahead in his path. The man of whom this friend wrote me deserved his death; if not for the specific act for which he was tried, then for other thoughts and acts which preceded that. The man was on the wrong road—a road of many and increasing evils. Death took him off the road at the right time, and gave him a better start in some other state of existence.

I must either believe this or deny the I Am God's power, wisdom or omnipresence. I must accept God's wisdom, power, love and presence on faith; or my own judgment on sight. As I know from experience that appearances are deceitful, and that my personal judgment must perforce be based almost entirely upon appearances, I prefer to hold fast my faith in the presence, power, wisdom and love of the God over all. Therefore I deny that this man suffered an untimely death for the vindictiveness and perjury of others; I believe he died as a result of a mental constitution and tendencies which are hidden from me, but not from the I Am. I believe it was the spirit of the I Am moving upon the face of his soul-deeps and saying, "Let there be light," which gave him his experiences and his particular form of death. And I believe his soul goes marching on to greater light—freed from the burdens of wrong habits of mind and body which were contracted in the old life of ignorance.

Oh, yes, it is easy to believe thus of one I never saw. It is not quite so easy to apply the same principle in the lives of those near and dear to me, and in my own life. But I aim to do it, even in the smallest details of living; and I am daily growing in the ability to acknowledge the I Am God in all my ways. I know this is the only way to live the new thought.

XVIII.

Immortal Thought.

I Am of every being is God, the only power, wisdom, will, mind; the only actor in all action; the only creator, disintegrator and recreator. The I Am of you is One, the Only One.

The I Am or ego or spiritual being of you is a thinker. All thinking is done by the one thinker— mortal thinking or immortal thinking.

Your body is an organization within you, the real you, the I Am, the thinker,—an organization within you of the thoughts you (the I Am or God) are thinking. Your body is the present conclusion of all the thoughts, good, bad or indifferent, true or untrue, mortal or immortal, which you have thought, unthought or rethought from the beginning of eternity; and hourly it is being changed by the new thoughts coming to you. The real, you does the thinking, recording conclusions in the body—which, mind you, is not you; nor does it even "contain" you; you are omnipresent, omnipotent, omniscient spirit or mind, and your body is within you. In you (God) it lives and moves and has its being, and by you (God) it is held together.

You have all-power to think all kinds of thoughts; and you use that power. You know you do—you know you think good thoughts, bad ones, mortal ones and immortal ones. Why question it? You think all kinds of thought. But that does not make you all kinds of a being. You are the One Being to whom all kinds of thinking are possible, just as you are a being to whom all sorts of acts are possible.

In their essence, thought and action are one. Are you a human being when you play on the piano and an animal when you sweep the floor? Are you a human being when you walk and a fish when you go swimming? Of course not. You are the One Being whatever you choose to do or think—you are God-being. One time you think mortal thoughts and the next time you think immortal thoughts (results always recording in your body) but always you are the same God-being.

And you feel all sorts of ways; but always you are you—the same One, God-being.

Your mortal thoughts are your thoughts of mortality—of death and all that leads to death—of sin, sickness, unhappiness, all that tends to discourage you from wanting to keep on living and thinking. Your immortal thoughts are your thoughts of life, activity,

140

love, joy—all those thoughts which make you want to live more. One thought differs from another but you go on forever, the same One God-being.

Your mystification all comes from confounding yourself with your thoughts; from thinking of your thought-built body as you—which it is not.

In its deepest analysis your body and all your thoughts are purely mortal thoughts, and only your real you, the thinker, is immortal. To be immortal is to be subject to no change—which is true of Life Principle only. To be mortal is to be subject to change and death—which is true of all thought, even thoughts of life, love, joy. All thoughts are fleeting and therefore "mortal" applies to them. Evil disappears before good thought, and "Good doth change to better, best."

The body is eternally changing—eternally receiving from the Self or spirit higher thought and eternally sloughing off lower thought. Body is mortal and will never be anything else. It will never cease to change; it will never cease to receive new thought and slough off back-number thought; it will never cease to "die daily." If it could for one hour cease this daily, hourly dying, this casting off thought which is out of date, it would die altogether.

Individual hanging on to dead thought is the cause of all old age and somatic death. The body instead of throwing off its dead and dying thought through its eliminative system, allows it to continue piling up in the body until death of the entire body comes as a relief. And the God-self goes on to new incarnations.

All bodily energy is the energy of live thought. Death comes to the body when dead thought preponderates. "Except ye become as a little child," whose daily dying is perfect, you shall continue to grow old and die the somatic death. A child hangs on to nothing. Every new thing charms it completely from the old, and its intense mental and physical activities keep the old moving out and off to make room for more of the new. Can you give any reason under the sun why human beings should not continue to live the child life and escape death of the body as a whole? There is no reason to be found in science, logic or nature; the one reason lies in our artificial living. We stuff the mind with unused knowledge; we stuff the body with twice to ten times the food we need (all food is thought, too); we glory in "owning" more things than we can possibly need or use; we spend our time straddling our possessions to keep others from using them; is it any wonder we become literally loaded down until our bodies are too cumbersome for any life more strenuous than that of the grave? Life to us is too real, too earnest; we want too much; and as long as we persist in living at this dying rate the grave will be our goal.

I said that in its last analysis all thought is mortal thought. This is true of formed thought, or thoughts. Thought substance is eternal; thought substance is "matter," without beginning or end; and matter in its original state is mind or spirit—the One Thinker and his thought material, one and indivisible. Thought substance is immortal, unchanging; but all forms of this thought substance are mortal, ever changing. Think of the ocean—the water is ever the same, but the waves, the forms assumed by the water, eternally change; so with thought substance and thought forms. The body being an organization of thought forms, of "mortal thoughts," must "die daily"; but that thought substance from which all its forms are made is immortal mind—is the God-self. Your body is simply a series or growing organization of fleeting eddies in your immortal God-self.

Too wonderful to grasp? Well, never mind—better not grasp it too tightly anyway—it might prove only another weight on your mind! Let the thought come and go in your consciousness, as waves come and go on the ocean; by and by you will "realize" that it is true— that you and the Father, body and soul, are all One and eternal. Just take it for granted, dearie, and love and be radiantly happy. So shall you use mortality to prove immortality.

I have said that the soul is not more than the body,
And I have said that the body is not more than the soul,
And nothing, not God, is greater to one than one's
self is,
And whoever walks a furlong without sympathy walks
to his own funeral drest in his shroud,
And I or you pocketless of a dime may purchase the
pick of the earth,
And to glance with an eye or show a bean in its pod
confounds the learning of all times,
And there is no trade or employment but the young
man following it may become a hero,
And there is no object so soft but it makes a hub for
the wheel'd universe,
And I say to any man or woman, Let your soul stand
cool and composed before a million universes.
And I say to mankind, Be not curious about God,
For I who am curious about each am not curious about
God.
(No array of terms can say how much I am at peace
about God and about death.)
I hear and behold God in every object yet understand
God not in the least,
Nor do I understand who there can be more wonderful
than myself.

—Walt Whitman.

XIX.

God in Person.

God is not *a* person; *he is all persons.*

"The Universe is One Stupendous Whole,
Whose body Nature is, and God the Soul."

This means that "Nature," which includes man, is the body of God; and God's body is to him what your body is to you—*a statement of beliefs which is eternally changing as experience teaches you more.*

The only body God has is your body and mine; the only brains he has are your brains and mine; the only experience he has is your experience and mine; the only judgment he has is your judgment and mine.

The only way God has of proving anything is through your experience and mine.

You have heard it said that you cannot teach a man anything he does not already know; that to educate a man is to draw out into consciousness that which is already within him. By his own experience and by the teaching of others he becomes conscious of the wisdom which was all the time within him. All knowledge is latent in God (the Whole) just as it is in you;

145

and God becomes conscious of what he knows by the same processes by which you become conscious. Your real self is God.

Watch yourself and you will see how God does things.

God is Wisdom. But Wisdom and knowledge are not identical. Knowledge is *Wisdom proved*—by the only proof, experience. All Wisdom is latent in God's soul, which is your soul and mine. God's Wisdom is *expressed* in his body, or "statement of beliefs," which is *your* body and mine.

God *knows* everything; but he *knows that he knows* only what he has proved through you and me, and all mankind and animalkind and vegetablekind.

"Some call it evolution; others call it God."

If God knew more he would not suffer through us. This is equivalent to saying if you and I knew more we would not suffer. *There is no you and I; there is only God.*

Evolution is simply God *coming into consciousness of himself and his wisdom.* Your body is a part of God's body; *your soul is God,* the One Life of all creation.

Do *you* wish to make his people suffer? Of course not. Do you wish to make yourself suffer? Of course you don't. *You are God, and you don't intentionally make anybody suffer unless you think you have to. The rest of the suffering you have not yet*

146

learned to avoid. In other words, God has not yet learned how to avoid it.

But evolution still evolutes, and sighing and sorrow are already fleeing before the dawn of Wisdom coming to itself. *God is learning how to enjoy himself in the flesh*—in your flesh and mine.

What *is* flesh? It is mind. God is learning to enjoy himself in his own mind, which is your flesh and mine. He keeps on thinking through you and me until his "statements of belief," his flesh body, bring only joy to all creation and uncreation.

Why did he make the ten commandments? Why do *you* lay down laws unto yourself? Because you *catch glimpses* of higher things than you have yet experienced, and you lay down laws which you mean to live up to.

But you don't always live up to those laws, do you? Why? Because your body is an organization of intelligent cells each of which has a will of its own. You catch a glimpse of the truth that Love is the Greatest Thing in the World; you lay down a commandment: "Thou shalt not be impatient or angry." Before a day has passed you catch yourself breaking your commandment—"you forgot." In other words, the most intelligent cells in your body recognized a beautiful truth and promulgated a new commandment for all the cells

147

to live by. But the less intelligent cells being still un-convinced of that beautiful truth, and being in a great majority, you did their will—you got mad.

Now God recognized through Moses most beautiful truths, and laid down laws to govern those who were as yet not intelligent enough to recognize the truths for themselves. For thousands of years God tried through these laws to make all the people see these truths. Thus his people evoluted—a little.

The God in Jesus caught a glimpse of still higher truth and laid down another law, that ye love one an-other. And still, after 2,000 years of that law, the people do not all see it, and very few of them obey.

A Moses or a Jesus recognizes truth so much greater than can be sensed by the common run of people, that it takes thousands of years of reiteration of that truth to make even a majority of the common run of people see it. It takes centuries of *evolution really* to convert the world to an Ideal conceived by a Jesus.

It takes you years of reiteration of your Ideal, and constant effort toward living up to it, before you can really convert your body to that Ideal.

In other words, *God* glimpses in Moses or Jesus a beautiful Ideal of himself; but it takes Him thousands and thousands of years to *work out* that Ideal, to evolute *all people* to the stage of wisdom and loving-kindness.

148

It is God's effort to work out his Ideals, which causes all suffering. This means that it is *your* effort to work out *your* Ideals, which causes all *your* suffering.

An Ideal impels change; the Established Order, in the Whole or a Part, *resents and resists* change; hence the pain. The spirit is willing but the flesh is established and refuses to change.

It was this Jesus had in mind when he said, *"Resist not evil."* The Established Order, the flesh, *resists change because it is too shortsighted to see that the change is good.* Because we are not yet convinced that *All* is Good and every change tends to greater good, we fight the change, more or less whole heartedly. We have within us the same high Ideals, the same backslidings and wars, revolutions and evolutions, the same joys and sorrows, that the children of Israel had, that the universe at large has had and is having. All history is the history of *your own thoughts.* Man is an infinite little cosmos.

Just as in history ignorance has warred against the Ideal and yet in the fullness of time the Ideal has had its way; so in yourself ignorance wars against the Ideal and may for a time seem to win, but eventually the Ideal has its way. A man in his ignorance may yield to "temptation" but *the results will take away the very temptation itself.* When a child's

149

fingers are *well* scorched it loses all desire to play with the fire.

There is no such thing as "ruining our lives forever." Every soul has *all eternity* in which to learn to live. Every soul is God—omnipresent, omniscient, or omnipotent *in potentiality*. And all eternity is its school term, all space its school ground. Death is simply a promotion ceremony, peculiar to the kindergarten classes. A "ruined" life is no more than a "ruined" problem on Tommy's slate—it is wiped off to give Tommy, who has been learning by his mistakes, a chance to do a better sum.

Be still and know that God and you are one, and all things shall be made plain.

XX.

How to Reach Heaven.

The subjective or emotional self is the best of servants but the worst of masters.

All the evil in the world results from transposing authority from objective to subjective, from letting emotion run away with conscience and reason.

All unpleasant reactions are due to the waste of energy which results from this transposition of authority.

The emotional or subjective self is the storehouse of personal power; the objective self is the director of that power. Happy results come from intelligent use of power. To give unbridled rein to the emotional self is like turning on the power of an automobile and then lying back and laughing—or weeping—whilst the auto runs its pace and kills or maims what comes in its way. The loud, hysterical giggle betrays that emotion is running away with the directing power, and that personal power is ebbing below the point of safety.

And the waste of power—the letting loose of more emotion than the occasion really calls for—is bound to produce its after effects of depression.

Depression of this sort is due to depletion of emotional energy, and disappears as the system recuperates —as more energy is stored.

Nearly all "blues" are caused by such reaction; energy is wasted in mental or physical agitation due to anger or fretting, or "righteous indignation," or excess of sympathy, or "having a good time"; and then we wonder why we are so blue. We go off and have a "good cry," which relaxes us, fall asleep after it, and wake up without the blues—and wonder why. More energy has been generated—that is all.

The secret of real enjoyment, of the kind from which there is no unpleasant reaction, lies in perfect control of the emotional nature; in so conserving your emotional power that it shall never be depleted beyond a certain definite point of poise, the point where there is plenty in well-controlled reserve.

When one first begins to find and maintain this state of poise he feels that he can never "have a good time" again—that he must repress all the fun and be glum and steady. But this is a mistaken idea, which will disappear as he gains control.

There are heights and depths and breadths of fun and joy which can never be touched except by the poised, controlled person.

It takes emotional energy to enjoy, and the greater

152

the store of energy the deeper the enjoyment, and the less of it is wasted in boisterous movements and noises.

One does not suppress his enjoyment of an incident; he suppresses unnecessary expressions of his enjoyment; and every such motion inhibited leaves him with that much more energy on hand with which to enjoy. In proportion as he ceases to slop his emotional power in loud laughs and unnecessary movements he deepens his power of enjoyment. Laughs are on the surface; real enjoyment is in the deeps of being. It is the surface slopping one must suppress, the waste of power, that he may become conscious of the real depths of enjoyment.

Impulsiveness' and nervousness are due to depleted emotional energy, and are invariably caused by letting the subjective, emotional self rule. So much energy is wasted in unnecessary emotionalism that there is not enough left to enjoy with—there are no depths. There comes to be a habitual waste of emotion over the most trivial things, and there is no reserve for the greater things which occasionally come. All due to excessive expression of emotion. People who have not learned to control their expressions of emotion have never even tasted full enjoyment.

The one cure for nervousness, impulsiveness, boister- -ous emotionalism of all sorts is to be still; cut off all unnecessary waste and let the reservoirs fill.

There are two kinds of "lively dispositions." One is the result of hysterical slopping over of energy without regard to the fact that the reservoirs of personal power are dangerously near the point of utter depletion. This sort of liveliness often ends in tears nearly always in depression. The other sort of "lively disposition" is the surface expression of full reservoirs. One is like the slopping of water from a shallow bowl, by shaking the bowl; the other is like the rippling of a clear lake —the depths are clear, still and happy, whilst the surface answers brightly and without waste, to the passing breezes of fun. The bowl of water is exhausted by its expressions of fun; the clear lake enjoys its ripples of laughter without wasting itself.

The larger the lake the larger the waves. The same breeze which causes a pond to ripple will cause Lake Michigan to toss in white-capped glee. The greater the length, breadth and depth the greater the waves; so, the greater the personal reservoir of emotional power the bigger the laugh of which it is capable. The loud laugh sometimes betrays the vacant mind and reservoirs; sometimes it betrays wide and deep and full ones; and by its ring the hearer can tell which. Who has not rippled in response to the musical, full, contagious loud laugh? And cringed at the sharp, hysterical loud laugh?

The musical laugh, loud or soft, invariably indicates

154

well stored reservoirs of emotional power and real enjoyment. The shrill unmusical laugh, the nervous laugh, loud or soft, invariably means nervous or emotional depletion, shallow reservoirs, and shallow enjoyment or none at all. Musical and unmusical speaking voices are other indications of these states of personal power. Smooth, graceful, intelligent gesticulations are yet other indications of full reservoirs; rough, jerky unnecessary motions indicating depletion.

The curtailing of wasteful laughs and motions is one of the most important things in life. Emotion is soul force, that which accomplishes all the great things of life as well as all the little things. Every human being has access to unlimited soul force, which is constantly flowing into him from the Universal Reservoir. But if he uses it as fast as it flows in—uses it in overdoing the small and least necessary things of life,—he has no power for the greater things every soul longs to do. How much power would the world get from the Niagara river if it were not for the great natural dam and reserve power at the falls? If you would do the great things you must see that your energy is not wasted in a steady stream of little things.

Every movement, every thought, uses a definite amount of emotional energy. Every inhibition of a movement or thought stream permits the higher rising of your reservoir; just as every stone added to a dam increases the reservoir and power behind it. There are enough good things to do and think in this beautiful world without dissipating our power in thoughtless activities, such as tapping our feet or fingers, rocking to and fro, giggling shrilly, and so on. Yes, we learn to do things by doing them; but do we want to do these useless things? Of course not. They are wasteful, unbeautiful

And we can learn to stop them by stopping them; and have so much deeper power with which to do the useful, beautiful things. A half hour a day used in simply being still, will add almost incredibly to the depth of our reservoirs. And every time we remember to inhibit an unnecessary rock or tap or fidget we add another depth to our power. This is all easily proved by a little practice.

Our energy is soul power, which is also wisdom. As our energy deepens our wisdom deepens also, and our sense of humor deepens. Soul power is love and wisdom, the One and Only Substance of which the individual is an inlet—a small or large inlet according as he lets the energy run out fast, or conserves it for large uses; according as he lets it run, or dams it for personal use.

There is plenty of soul power for everything—yes. But it takes time to build a dam; and the man who lets loose his whole Niagara Falls of emotion upon trivial occasions will have to spend most of his time in patching his dam. And the man who dribbles all his power in thoughtless and useless acts has no power behind his Niagara.

Do you see that self-control is the key of heaven? And the time to use it is now, the place here. "Earth's crammed with heaven" waiting to be conserved to individual uses. Love, power, wisdom is flowing through you into expression—don't let it flow too fast—don't waste it in thoughtless, foolish expression. Cut off the wastes; use the power in wise directions, and let the tide rise within you. Thus shall you come to the great things you would do, and behold within you shall be the power to do them with joy; and there shall be no aftermath of depression.

This is heaven—the highest heaven for the deepest soul.

And the door is open for everybody.

*   *   *   *   *   *

Vital energy is soul energy—love-power and wisdom mixed—L^2W^2.

The body is a generator of vital or soul energy.

Heaven and hell are states of bodily being. The body full of vital or soul energy—L^2W^2—experiences heaven.

The body depleted of its soul energy lives in hell—carried there by riotous living, by wasting its vital or soul energy.

I know I am august,
I do not trouble my spirit to vindicate itself or be
    understood,
I see that the elementary laws never apologize.
(I reckon I behave no prouder than the level I plant
    my house by, after all.)

I exist as I am, that is enough,
If no other in the world be aware I sit content,
And if each and all be aware I sit content.

One world is aware and by far the larger to me, and
    that is myself,
And whether I come to my own to-day or in ten thou-
    sand or ten million years,
I can cheerfully take it now, or with equal cheerfulness
    I can wait.

My foothold is tenon'd and mortis'd in granite,
I laugh at what you call dissolution,,
And I know the amplitude of time.
                                    —Walt Whitman.

XXI.

A Look at Heredity.

No evolutionist can overlook heredity, nor underestimate it. He believes that every generation comes in on the shoulders of its predecessors, and he fully appreciates the value of good predecessors. The world's pride of ancestry is not so foolish as it might appear. The more intelligence and culture my forbears had the greater my possibilities. There are no breaks in the law of growth or evolution or heredity, though the casual observer often fancies there are.

Every human being comes into the world as an "acme of things accomplished" by his ancestors, and he is an "encloser of things to be" accomplished by himself and his progenitors.

But who are my ancestors? Let me tell you that Ralph Waldo Emerson and Jesus of Nazareth are more directly my ancestors than many of those whom the world calls my great-grandfathers. There is a spiritual and mental kinship through which we inherit. There are spiritual and mental relationships to which we all owe far more of our goodness and greatness than

159

can be traced to those of blood tie. In rare instances only do these spiritual and mental relationships exist within the line of blood relationship.

The world does well to be proud of its ancestry; but it does better when it appreciates its spiritual ancestry. Think you that the poor little waif owes a larger inheritance to the woman who bore it and deserted it, than to the foster parents who nurtured it in love and wisdom?

Our blood relations are not the only relations from whom we inherit; neither when we are born do we cease to inherit. There is One Father of us all, and the oft-repeated statement that we are all brothers and sisters is no fanciful one. The "fatherhood of God and brotherhood of man" is fact; and the man who thinks he is limited by the ignorance of his blood relations is himself an ignoramus. If his blood relations are not to his liking, let him draw a new inheritance from the world's greatest and best. They, too, are his ancestors.

And mark this: Not only does the son inherit from his fathers of blood or spirit tie, but many a father inherits from the son that which the son has gained from other sources than those of blood relationship. Inheritance by blood tie is not a stream, the outlet of which can rise no higher than its source. It is a sort of hydraulic ram. through which life may be coaxed to almost any height of culture and refinement.

I have heard it said that culture is "the soul of knowledge—the essence of right living" inherited from our ancestors. Where did they get it? I will tell you where; they got it by persistence in the same sort of practices which are decried—by "wresting, by force," the knowledge, wealth and dominion of others; by generations of "monastic seclusion," much of it enforced by others whose turn it was to "wrest by force"; by generations of "rigid self-control"; by hours and days and years of prayer, which is simply a phase of "going into the silence"; and, yes, and even by "breathing like a filthy, crazy Yoga"—though much of the breathing was forced by strenuous endeavors to get away from the raging hordes whose wealth or daughters they were stealing. The Spirit of Evolution which is running this universe is very cunning in devices for inducing self-culture.

Full breathing, going into the silence, affirmations, etc., are not new methods of self-culture. They are as old and their practice as universal as life itself. But heretofore their practice has been in the main compulsory. Humanity had to be persecuted, starved, hunted into breathing, exercising, praying—had to be forced to develop body, soul and wits by using them.

The present generation inherits the wisdom gained through their efforts. Not the least of its inheritance

161

lies in its wits developed to the point of seeing that for self-development ten minutes of voluntary deep breathing is preferable to an all-day chase to save one's neck; that a half hour of intelligent silence is worth more than the three and four hour "wrestlings with the Lord" such as our great-grandfather John Wesley—and many of his inheritors—practiced regularly.

Herein lies the great difference between our ancestors and us: They were by conditions compelled to self-culture; whilst we, their inheritors, are making intelligent use of it.

Through evolution we are learning to conserve energy. Our ancestors spent all their time—perforce—in half-unconscious physical exercise and breathings; we spend a few minutes a day in intelligent exercise and breathing, and conserve our forces for mental and spiritual uses.

And without them we should be minus the intelligence to do this. Humanity is a solidarity—on the square; and without the work of his ancestors none shall be made perfect.

But it is by the work of his ancestors that man stands on to-day's pinnacle. What they learned to do by labored effort and mainly under compulsion, we do by instinct.

It is by man's work to-day on this pinnacle, that his

great-grandchildren shall be brought forth on yet higher pinnacles, with yet higher instinctive knowledge.

Take the most cultured person you know; trace his ancestry and tell me where his culture began. You cannot do it. Go clear back to William the Conqueror if you will; thus far you may call his ancestors cultured, but even so their culture, all the way back, is a descending scale of boorishness in comparison with what we twentieth century folk call culture. And we must hark back of William for the beginning of his culture. William the Conqueror was the illegitimate son of Robert the Devil. Did culture begin with Robert? And the mother of William was a miller's daughter. Is she the mother of all culture? Robert the Devil was the third earl of Normandy; which means that his grandfather was an ordinary everyday scrub who probably murdered somebody particularly obnoxious to the king and was rewarded with an earldom. Did he bequeath "the soul of knowledge, the essence of right living," to William the Conqueror and his exclusive progeny? If so, where did he get it? His own grandfather and the ancestors of the poor miller's daughter roamed the same woods, fought the same battles, hunted the same beasts and men, and gnawed the same bones. Where did the ancestors of Robert the Devil pick up the "soul of knowledge"? And what were the

163

miller's ancestors doing whilst Robert's grandfathers cornered the "essence of right living"? For I warrant you that William's miller's-daughter-mother was less of a stranger to the "soul of knowledge, the essence of right living" than was that devil of a Robert.

Yes, there are many people who are educated but not cultured. But their progeny will brag of their culture. For what is in one generation mere education, or "monastic seclusion," or "rigid self-control," or "going into the silence," or "breathing like a filthy, crazy Yoga," is by time and unconscious cerebration transmuted into pure "culture." And if any of us lack culture you may depend upon it our ancestors, by blood and spirit, are numbered among those who failed to "wrest by force" the very things decried as uncultured.

All life is education; and time transmutes education into culture, "the soul of knowledge, the essence of right living."

Not a human effort but is necessary to the development of the soul of knowledge. Not a Yoga breath, not an hour of silence, not a moment of rigid self-control, not a day of hard labor, not a sound or movement or cry of joy or sorrow or rage or despair,—not one but has helped to free the soul of knowledge. Not one could have been dispensed with without leaving culture less cultured than it is.

164

The difference between education and culture is the difference between the daily drill at the piano and the finished musical expression of a Paderewski. Education comes first and without it there can be no culture. Education is the work of TODAY; whilst culture is the soul of well used yesterdays. Why exalt the well used yesterdays to the disparagement of today's opportunities?

Inheritance is wealth left us by sanguine and spiritual relations gone before. It is capital left us, to be increased by just such "wresting by force" as some people condemn. Who is the more valuable to the human race:—he who parades his inheritance as he received it or he who adds to it his own efforts at self-culture?

. Don't be a Chinaman and kow-tow eternally to heredity. Be an Individual and improve heredity. If your inheritance was poor make it better; if it was good make it better. The world's culture is only just beginning; get busy helping it along. That is the important thing.

Do it now.

Idealist.

Lo, I am Skeptic! neither bind
Science nor Bible on my mind.

All things I hold in flux; the Good,
Fore-running Dream paints to my mood.

The sweet Ideal is more to me
Than any man's philosophy.

The Books no man may surely know,
Science is changeful, doubtful, so,

Doubter, my faith is more than most,
My Dream of Best I give my trust.

In it I think Divinity
Speaks surest to the core of me.

By night clear fire, by day bright cloud,
Music of Sphere, soul-sweet, brain-loud.

Heart-thrilling, lures me on, the God
Floating before with smile and nod.

The best I dream, my faith tells me,
Will come to live as grows a tree,

As breaks a day, and life must hold
A fact each dream a hope can mould.

—J. William Lloyd.

XXII.

Critic and Criticised.

"I don't want to be criticised."

"But you want to learn, don't you? You surely are not satisfied that you know it all."

"Oh, of course I want to learn, but I want to learn by myself. I would rather be wrong than be criticised. I hate to be told how to do things. I want to find out for myself."

Solomon the Wise reasons not thus. Solomon prayed for wisdom above all things, and in receiving wisdom he received all else.

The man who thinks he would rather be wrong than be criticised is for the time being a moral coward and no Solomon. He values his "feelings" of the moment above wisdom. He does not want wisdom and knowledge above all things; he wants what wisdom and knowledge he can gain without the sacrifice of his feeling of self-complacency. He is complacent as long as his friend says to him, "You are a good fellow, a very admirable fellow"; he feels good as long as he thinks his friend considers him wise;

167

he expands and smiles, and works away in his own good way.

In his moments of confidence he will tell his friend that Wisdom and Knowledge are the greatest things in the universe; that we grow only by the acquisition of Wisdom and Knowledge; that growth is Life, and Life is Love or God. He will enthuse a bit and tell you Wisdom is God, the One Desirable One; and that by growing in wisdom man becomes conscious of his divinity.

Just here his friend, who is a prosy, practical sort of fellow, interrupts him. "See here, Smith," he says, "you are not running this branch of your business quite right. You just ought to see how Thomson does that sort of thing."

He gets no farther; Smith freezes instantly, and Jones's confidences catch the vibrations. Smith is "so sensitive, you know"—he would rather not know anything about better methods, than to stand the shock of a criticism. Jones talks about the weather a bit, and departs.

Smith continues to think he desires wisdom above all things.

He does n't. He desires above all things to have his bump of approbativeness smoothed.

He fails to know himself. And he will not learn

himself, because he refuses all truth which does not make him "feel" good.

He shuts himself off from a thousand avenues by which wisdom is trying to reach him.

It is said our enemies are our best friends. Emerson bids us listen to them and learn of them.

Burns exclaims:—

> "O wad some power the giftie gie us
> To see oursels as ithers see us!
> It wad frae mony a blunder free us
> And foolish notion."

Our critics are answering Love's attraction to free us from blunders and foolish notions.

Why not? Why resent a criticism? We are all members of "One Stupendous Whole." Why resent and refuse another's suggestion? It is our own suggestion, drawn by our own affirmed love for wisdom and knowledge.

We don't understand ourselves; we don't trust our surroundings. We say we want wisdom above all things; we want to understand. In our heart of hearts we do love wisdom above all things; therefore we attract it through all avenues.

It is our soul's love for wisdom and knowledge which attracts to us the criticisms of friend and foe.

If we really believed that we attract what we receive;

that "our own" comes to us; that all things are working together to gratify our soul's desires;—if we really believed all this we would meet criticism in a friendly spirit, with senses alert to find the kernel of wisdom it is bringing us.

To resent a criticism is to re-send, to send away, a bit of knowledge your soul has been praying for. All because your bump of approbativeness has an abnormal appetite for prophecies of "smooth things."

But to re-send a criticism is not to get rid of it. It comes back to you over and over, and perhaps every time in a little ruder form.

If you speak softly to a friend and he fails to hear, you repeat in a louder tone; if he is very deaf you holler, and perhaps touch his shoulder to gain his attention.

All creation is alive, and pursues the same tactics. When you resent, re-send, a criticism, Creation sends it back at you a little more emphatically. If you still resent it Creation puts still more force into repeated sendings. She keeps this up, in answer to your own semi-conscious desire for wisdom and knowledge, until by some hook or crook you take the kernel of knowledge contained in that criticism. Then Creation smiles and lets you alone—on that line.

The way to avoid Creation's kicks is to accept her

hints as they come to you in the form of friendly criticism or suggestion.

Not all criticisms are true in their entirety, but every one contains somewhere a suggestion by which you may profit—by which you may grow in wisdom and knowledge.

Don't let that one little bump of approbativeness make you re-send that knowledge—and bring down Creation's kicks to drive it home.

But don't get the idea that that little round nub of approbation is "bad." He is not. He is a good and useful member of your family, and deserves to be well fed and cared for and respected.

But feed him so well on your own good opinions that he will not sulk and kick if he does n't receive unlimited taffy from others. Get away up high in your own opinion. Know yourself a god, unique, indispensable to Creation. You have powers and wisdom and knowledge not possessed by anybody else in the world. Nobody who ever lived or ever will is any better or any more of a god than you are.

Neither is anybody less good or less of a god than you. We are different—that is all. Every man has his individual goodnesses and his peculiar point of view —no better than yours, but different.

It takes every man in the world to see all sides of anything, or anybody.

Every individual who is at all wise wants to see all sides of things. The only chance he has of doing this is to look at things from other people's points of view, as well as his own; to put himself in other people's places; to see as others see; to vibrate with the other fellow—who sees another side of the same thing.

Listen to your critic. See yourself as he sees you. He is your best friend, drawn in answer to your soul's cry for more wisdom and knowledge. Be friends with him. Hush the clamor of approbativeness with your own high affirmations of your goodness and worth— hush the clamor and listen. The spirit in you will separate the chaff from the wheat of the criticism; a smiling little "Poof!" will blow away the chaff; and your soul will expand and increase in stature by assimilating the wheat.

XXIII.

The Nobility.

We always come in contact with the people we live and think up to. If you are not satisfied with present environment it can be changed by making your very best of it, and in the meantime fitting yourself mentally, physically and in deportment, for the sort of people you want. Get ready for 'em.

And see you waste no energy in impatience over having to wait a long time.

It takes mental and physical culture and gracious deportment to fit you for the sort of friends you want.

There is no place in life which does not offer plenty of advantages for the cultivation of all these things, but especially for the cultivation of a gracious deportment. You may depend that if you can be lovely and gracious to "common people," who may ruffle your feathers the wrong way, you will be at home if a duchess happens along. Duchesses, you know, belong to the class of people who make a study and lifelong practice of being lovely and gracious. I am talking about real duchesses

173

now—not the kind that get rich quick and marry a title without having the real qualifications of nobility.

Somebody has said that the world is divided into two classes, the civil and the uncivil. The hall-mark of real nobility is the habit of being civil to the uncivil. No better place to acquire this gentle art than living among the uncivil. The youth who finds himself among the uncivil and who proceeds to cultivate uppishness and contempt for his associates; who "looks down" on those with whom he is compelled to associate; who tries to be "superior" and to impress others with his superiority,—such an one is forever fixing himself in the class of the uncivil—where duchesses don't grow.

You *are* what you are. Time spent in trying to "impress" people is worse than wasted. Be your gracious self, and honor not only your father and your mother but your next door neighbor and your next door neighbor's kitchen maid if you want to develop the qualities that will fit you for the sort of associates you want—members of the really truly nobility.

Cultivate your brains, dearie; cultivate your body; cultivate your soul; all to the best of your ability. But above all and in all and through all cultivate the mental and physical deportment of the truly noble. Belong always to the civil class and practice civility eternally upon the uncivil as well as upon the civil.

When a brawling enemy followed Pericles home one dark night, with intent to injure him, Pericles sent his own servant with a lantern to light the man home again. Pericles did not descend from his own class to pay his uncivil enemy in his own coin.

Go thou and cultivate Pericles and thine own high self. Then shall all desirable associates seek you, instead of you having to seek them.

Greater credit belongs to him who sees the real nobility through the housemaid's dress and manner, than to him who recognizes it in silk and velvet voice.

We are all members of the nobility, all descended through Adam and Eve, who never saw silk nor made salaams. All are sons and daughters of the Most High.

Don't be fooled into contempt and incivility by our masquerade costumes; and don't value some of our gowns above ourselves—or yourself.

L' Envoi.

When earth's last picture is painted,
* And the tubes are twisted and dried,*
When the oldest colors have faded,
* And the youngest critic has died,*
We shall rest—and, faith, we shall need it—
* Lie down for an aeon or two,*
Till the Master of All Good Workmen
* Shall set us to work anew.*

And those that were good shall be happy—
* They shall sit in a golden chair;*
They shall splash at a ten-league canvas
* With brushes of comet's hair.*
They shall find real saints to draw from—
* Magdalene, Peter, and Paul;*
They shall work for an age at a sitting,
* And never get tired at all.*

And only the Master shall praise us,
* And only the Master shall blame;*
And no one shall work for money,
* And no one shall work for fame;*
But each for the joy of the working,
* And each in his separate star,*
Shall draw the thing as he sees it,
* For the God of things as they are.*

—Rudyard Kipling.

176

Printed in the United States
77423LV00002B/63